Also by Nina Shandler

The Complete Guide and Cookbook for
Raising Your Child As a Vegetarian

Holiday Sweets Without Sugar

Homemade Mixes for Instant Meals the Natural Way

How to Make All the Meat You Eat Out of Wheat

Ways of Being Together: A Guide for Couples

Yoga for Pregnancy and Birth:
A Guide for Expectant Parents

The Marriage and Family Book

ESTROGEN: THE NATURAL WAY

ESTROGEN: THE NATURAL WAY

Over 250 Easy and Delicious Recipes for Menopause

NINA SHANDLER

Villard
New York

Library of Congress Cataloging-in-Publication Data
Shandler, Nina.
Estrogen: the natural way : over 250 easy and delicious
recipes for menopause / Nina Shandler.
p.   cm.
Includes index.
ISBN 0-375-75141-6
1. Menopause—Complications—Diet therapy—Recipes.   2. Menopause—
Nutritional aspects.   3. Middle-aged women—Nutrition.
4. Soyfoods—Therapeutic use.   5. Flaxseed—Therapeutic use.
I. Title.
RG186.S6613   1997
618.1'750654—dc21   96-39670

24689753
First Paperback Edition
Book design by Debbie Glasserman

To the most thoroughly good people I know:
my mother, Mabel Silverberg, who has stayed sprightly
on a diet of kind thoughts,
and
my father, Carl Silverberg, who has nurtured
my confidence since the day I was born

Motivated by Menopause

During my first year of menopause, my life and my body changed.

Just as I was about to embark on my second adulthood, Manju, my older daughter, began her first. She graduated from Bennington College and moved to New York City. So, suddenly, she was no longer calling our house "home." She was an artist, living on her own. As she prepared for her first show in the big city, she made a doll. Pleased with her production, she phoned me. "Mom, I made this doll. It's sort of weird. Sort of creepy. Ugly. I love it."

I went to New York. I walked into Manju's apartment and entered her room. The doll sat in a corner. I sat down with the doll. I looked at her face. I could look at nothing else. Standing at the door of her room, Manju explained, "I've been thinking about making her for a long time. She's a doll who got left in an attic. She grew old. She aged. Do you like her?" I stared at this tiny vulnerable being—my daughter's creation. Her face was lined. Her forehead was furrowed. Her hair was thin. Her dress was faded. I touched her feet. Soft as a baby's, yet they looked as if they had traveled through a century. I held her little, frail, withered hands. I felt as if she had received my touch, as though she were grateful for the acceptance. I said, "Manju. She's wonderful. She's so wonderful." Manju told me, "My roommates think she's scary." I said, "She's just old." I held the doll and felt as if I were holding myself. I realized, "I have to nurture my own body the way I once nurtured my babies."

This book began as a personal project in my own menopausal self-care. My extreme hot flashes had convinced me I needed estrogen. When I couldn't tolerate hormone replacement pills, I investigated and discovered the existence of plant estrogens. I changed my diet. Along the way, I learned to love cooking for myself as much as I once loved making Mickey Mouse pancakes for my daughters, Manju and Sara.

One evening, my dear friend and neighbor Margaret stopped by. I was eating one of my new inventions—a chocolate pudding. "Eat this," I insisted. She complied. She savored every bite. She offered her culinary critique: "I love it." Then I broke the news: "It's tofu." She said, "Really! Give me the recipe."

My husband, Michael, looked up from reading Gail Sheehy's *New Passages* and commented, "You should write a book about plant estrogens." At that moment, this book was conceived.

To ensure that the book would be healthy, honest, and medically responsible, I enlisted the aid of three nutritionally oriented physicians. Their explanation of the well-researched estrogenic potential of food follows.

Next comes the story of my personal adventure in menopausal self-care, how I developed a workable, enjoyable dietary program for my own needs.

Before launching into recipes, I describe estrogen-rich plant foods—what they are, where to find them, and how to use them.

Finally, I share more than 250 recipes, all tested in my own kitchen.

I truly hope this book helps you to nurture yourself safely through the second half of your life.

Acknowledgments

My list of people to thank begins with those who saw the possibilities for this project and nurtured it along the way:

Agnes Birnbaum, my agent, gave her all to this endeavor from the moment of our first conversation. She shepherded my proposal through the publishing world and shielded me from discouragement. At every turn, she cared for me as well as for my work.

Annik La Farge, my editor at Villard, saw the potential of this project and enabled me to tap it. She gave me the confidence to tell my story in my own voice, and she had the objectivity to tell me when that voice became breathless. She has been quick, smart, enthusiastic, and supportive—everything an author could want from an editor.

Betsy Rapoport at Times Books was the first editor at Random House to see the proposal for this book. She passed it on to Annik, at Villard, but never abandoned it. She generously read the manuscript and gave valued suggestions.

Creating every book is a team effort. The entire Villard staff has rallied around this project. David Rosenthal, the publisher, lent his support throughout the entire process. Always pleasant and patient,

Melissa Milsten steered it along the route from manuscript to finished book. Dan Rembert, the art director, Mary Ann Smith, the cover artist, and Debbie Glasserman designed an aesthetically appealing book from cover to cover. Sybil Pincus oversaw the production editing with respect for my meaning. Emily Pearl copyedited the manuscript with a meticulous eye for every important detail. Kirsten Raymond, my talented publicist, took on this project with unbounded enthusiasm, guiding and soothing me during my most fretful media moments. I'm grateful to the entire energetic organization.

Michael Shandler, my husband, gave me the idea for this book. During its creation, he has tasted every recipe and read every line. In many ways this book is his baby—he conceived it and guided it through both the writing and the taste-testing process.

Barry Elson, M.D., Joyce Duncan, M.D., and Samuel Gladstone, M.D., accepted my proposal of partnership with enthusiasm. They gave this book credibility and contributed their expertise. Barry's extensive understanding of natural alternatives to hormone replacement therapy, Joyce's knowledge of women's health issues, and Sam's responsible questioning of evidence combined to create a careful and helpful analysis of the medical and nutritional value of plant estrogens. Perhaps best of all, we had fun. Our working relationships have been nothing but good.

Alicia Landman, M.D., provided thoughtful feedback on the first draft. Albey Reiner, Ph.D., helped me grapple with the project's feasibility.

In addition to these primary players, I also want to thank others. My wonderful children, Sara and Manju, deserve thanks for tolerating my estrogenic obsession. Jeff and Di Krauth, owners of Beyond Words Bookshop, made helpful title suggestions. My good friends—Margaret and Philip Gosselin, Martin and Melly Bock, Mary and Herb Bernstein, Joan and Rob Brandt, Laurie Pearlman, Ervin Staub, Ann Berliner, Vicky Elson, and Gavin Harrison—offered encouragement and praised my recipes.

Contents

Preface: Motivated by Menopause   ix

Acknowledgments   xi

Introduction: The Estrogen-Diet Connection   xv
  by Barry Elson, M.D., Joyce Duncan, M.D., and Samuel Gladstone, M.D.

  1 Searching for Safe Passage: My Story   3
  2 The Plant Estrogen Pantry   27
  3 Munchables   41
  4 Breakfast   73
  5 Spreads and Breads   106
  6 Soups   132
  7 Condiments   150
  8 Salads and Side Dishes   161
  9 Pasta and Rice   186
 10 Main Dishes   202
 11 Desserts   230

Sources of Ingredients   273
References   275
Index   283

Introduction

The Estrogen-Diet Connection

by Barry Elson, M.D., Joyce Duncan, M.D., and Samuel Gladstone, M.D.

Women need estrogen. But how much estrogen do they need? And for how long? Medical science cannot answer these questions with certainty. While a growing body of research suggests that estrogen may protect hearts and bones, other research points to possible increased risk of breast cancer from overexposure to estrogen. Nature has programmed women's bodies to produce less estrogen as they grow older. We do not fully understand why estrogen levels diminish naturally. We do not know what levels of estrogen will benefit women without endangering them.

This uncertainty leaves women with a distressing dilemma: Estrogen pills appear to protect many women against some of the discomforts and diseases of aging, but these same pills may place them in harm's way. Medical research indicates that to secure the long-term benefits of conventional hormone replacement therapy, long-term use may be required. With long-term use seems to come increased risk of breast cancer. Amid the confusion, women are looking for ways to replace lost estrogen without endangering themselves—for ways to maintain the health of their hearts and bones while protecting themselves from breast cancer.

The estrogen decision is a medically complex individual choice—one not to be taken lightly. Estrogen and progesterone may be helpful to some women, but these same drugs may be harmful to others. For some, they alleviate discomfort. Hot flashes cease. Emotions stabilize. Languishing libidos reawaken. Minds sharpen. For others, hormone replacement therapy increases discomfort. Nausea, headaches, anxiety, irritability, moodiness, abdominal bloating, fluid retention, vaginal discharge, rashes, itching, nasal congestion, depression, breast tenderness, and increased appetite may accompany the ingestion of estrogen and progesterone. While hormone replacement therapy appears to decrease the risk of heart disease and osteoporosis, other health problems may result from its use. In *The Estrogen Decision,* Susan Lark, M.D., points out that increased risk of liver and gallbladder disease, high blood pressure, blood clotting, diabetes, uterine fibroid tumors, endometriosis, and, most important, breast cancer may be side effects of pharmaceutical estrogen. Isaac Schiff, M.D., chief of obstetrics and gynecology at Massachusetts General Hospital, sums up the predicament clearly: "Basically, you're presenting women with the possibility of increasing the risk of getting breast cancer at age sixty in order to prevent a heart attack at age seventy and a hip fracture at age eighty. How can you make that decision . . . ?" The pros and cons of hormone replacement therapy weigh heavily on all menopausal women.

Most women believe that taking estrogen pills is the only way to obtain the health benefits of estrogen after menopause. Few know that plants contain different forms of estrogen. These plant estrogens—called *phytoestrogens, isoflavones,* or *lignans*—appear to provide estrogenic effects while reducing the risk of breast cancer. Soy and flaxseed contain substantially larger quantities of plant estrogens than other foods. Exciting new research suggests that consuming soy and flaxseed may provide estrogenic benefits while decreasing the risk of breast cancer.

Not long ago, any suggestion that dietary changes might provide health benefits comparable to medication would have sounded like the ravings of a health-food fringe. Today, research has changed that perception. The beneficial effects of diet on heart disease are now widely acknowledged. New studies point to the possibility that certain cancers, as well as osteoporosis, may also be affected by diet. The *New England Journal of Medicine,* the *Journal of the National Cancer Institute, Lancet,* the *Journal of Steroid Biochemistry and Molecular Biology, Maturitas: Journal of Climacteric and Postmenopause, Cancer Research,* and the *British Medical Journal* are just a few of the prestigious medical journals that have published articles pointing to the potential protective effects and health benefits of soy and/or flaxseed.

In this important book, Nina Shandler shows women how to reap the potential benefits of plant estrogens. By taking her own self-care seriously, she has paved a path for other women. Using reputable medical and nutritional research, she has put an estrogenic dietary program within the grasp of every menopausal and postmenopausal woman. By clearly charting how much soy and flaxseed have demonstrated specific health benefits, Shandler enables women to plan their diets to meet their own needs. Her nondogmatic approach encourages women to use estrogen-rich foods as either an alternative or complementary form of medicine. Women who wish to avoid hormone replacement therapy will find Shandler's personal story and her approach reassuring. Women who decide to take hormone replacement therapy will find a measure of comfort as they examine the potential breast cancer–protective benefits of soy and flaxseed. Best of all, the author's estrogen-rich recipes are fun, fast, and delicious. We can personally attest to their mouthwatering goodness. Everything from Shandler's kitchen, from breakfast to dessert, tastes like pure indulgence. Women will not have to sacrifice their taste buds to comply with this diet plan!

☰ THE MANY FACES OF ESTROGEN

Before sitting down to consume daily doses of dietary estrogen, women need some questions answered. If estrogen is estrogen, then what difference does it make whether it comes from pills or plants? Why is it that the estrogen in hormone replacement therapy places women at greater risk for breast cancer, while the estrogen in soy and flaxseed protects women from breast cancer?

Contrary to popular belief, estrogen has many forms. Some appear to increase the risk of breast cancer, others to reduce it. Some estrogens are produced by the body, and some are found in animal foods, some in the environment, and some in plants.

Within the body, estrogen takes three primary forms. A growing body of research indicates that two forms promote cancer and one appears to protect against cancer. When women take conventional pharmaceutical estrogen replacement therapy, they ingest the two cancer-implicated forms of estrogen. When women eat soy and flaxseed, they consume weak plant estrogens that may actually guard against breast cancer.

▧ ESTROGEN: CANCER PROMOTER OR CANCER PROTECTION?

To understand how estrogen can both promote cancer and protect against cancer requires untangling its multiple forms. The estrogens produced by the body come in different strengths, comparable to the octane levels of gasoline. Estradiol, the highest octane, is eighty times more potent than estriol, the weakest. Estrone, the midgrade octane, is twelve times stronger than estriol. All three grades do largely the same work. All keep hearts healthy, bones strong, skin young, and vaginal linings moist. All permeate cells from head to toe, beginning at conception. Different forms of estrogen are more or less active at different stages of life.

In childhood, women's bodies produce small quantities of estrogen. Then in adolescence, the ovaries activate, producing twenty times as much estradiol as in childhood. As menopause approaches, estradiol production slows. In menopause, the ovaries stop producing estradiol, but other organs and tissues, primarily the adrenal glands and fat cells, generate limited amounts of the midgrade estrone for as long as twenty years.

Both the estradiol generated by the ovaries and the estrone manufactured by the adrenals, fat, and other tissues have cancer-promoting potential. It seems to be largely the responsibility of the liver to regulate estrogen, to provide protection from the estradiol and estrone. The healthy liver appears to transform estradiol and estrone into a benign mix by changing a portion of the estradiol and estrone into estriol. This transformation seems, at least in part, to disarm the cancer threat. Systematic and intensive investigation by H. P. Lemon, M.D., reported in the *Journal of the American Medical Association,* indicates that the balance of all three estrogens may be a key to lowering breast cancer risk. Evidence suggests that if the balance is thrown off—if the proportion of estradiol and estrone outweighs the proportion of estriol too heavily—the risk of breast cancer increases. Given this research, some nutritionally oriented physicians prescribe an unconventional form of hormone replacement therapy. These pills include all three forms of estrogen in proportions adjusted to mimic a low-risk premenopausal balance.

Nevertheless, the earlier women start menstruating and the later they stop—in other words, the longer their exposure to strong estrogens— the greater their likelihood of developing breast cancer. Prolonged exposure to strong estrogens contributes to greater breast cancer risk.

Excess weight appears to endanger women in much the same way. Fat cells produce estrone. Overweight women are exposed to a lifetime of strong estrogen, increasing their risk of breast cancer.

There is another way women prolong their exposure to the two strong cancer-implicated estrogens, estradiol and estrone: They take estrogen replacement pills.

Estrogen replacement proved risky to our mothers. A generation ago, doctors believed estrogen replacement would keep our mothers eternally youthful. Unfortunately, the enthusiastic experiment in staying young forever backfired: Estrogen replacement resulted in a tenfold increase in uterine cancer.

Researchers designed a new regime. Women in the 1990s take progesterone to limit the devastation wrought by the two strong estrogens. The currently advised hormone replacement regimen—the addition of progesterone—has eliminated the increase in uterine cancer. Some concern now exists, however, that progesterone may also limit the heart-helpful effects of estrogen even while it seems to increase protection from osteoporosis.

Given past misjudgments, continued wavering, and periodic reassessments, many women feel insecure about their doctors' advice regarding hormones. They wonder if another deadly cancer risk accompanies their prescription medicine.

Breast cancer is the greatest concern, and women have good reason to worry. Breast cancer plagues one in eight women at some time in their lives. Christiane Northrup, M.D., a gynecologist and the author of *Women's Bodies, Women's Wisdom,* explains: "Since breast tissue has estrogen receptors in it and is estrogen sensitive, it makes sense that in a woman at risk for breast cancer, estrogen replacement therapy (estradiol and estrone) could start a tumor growing that might otherwise have been dormant."

In the summer of 1995, these fears found more confirmation. Harvard researchers documented the long-term effects of hormone replacement therapy on 120,000 women. They found that estrogen replacement pills increased the risk of breast cancer by 30 percent. With the addition of progesterone, the risk increased to 40 percent. The study's primary researcher, Graham Colditz, offered clear advice: "Don't take hormones for a long time if you can avoid it."

The truly critical question is this: Can women replenish their diminishing estrogen supplies with a potentially cancer-protective form of estrogen rather than a potentially cancer-promoting form?

The simple answer to this question is yes. Potentially cancer-protective estrogen can be found in food.

PLANT ESTROGENS: SOY AND FLAXSEED

The easiest, simplest, healthiest, safest way to ingest estrogen is to eat it. Many foods—especially soy and flaxseed—contain plant estrogens. In 1990 a pioneering study published in the *British Journal of Medicine* demonstrated the estrogenic effects of soy and flaxseed. The average age of the women chosen for the study was fifty-nine. None had taken any form of hormone replacement therapy. The researchers supplemented the women's usual diet with 45 grams of soy flour (about

6 tablespoons) or 25 grams of flaxseed (about 2 tablespoons) daily. These women began the study well entrenched in postmenopausal symptoms. To measure the estrogenic effects of soy and flaxseed, the researchers analyzed their vaginal mucous. At the beginning of the study, the vaginal linings of all the women showed the markings of estrogen deprivation. Without making any other lifestyle changes, the women showed real, positive, quantifiable estrogenic changes in six weeks. Their vaginal secretions regenerated, resembling those of premenopausal women. After they stopped the soy or flaxseed regimen, their vaginal moisture remained elevated for two weeks. After eight weeks, their vaginal secretions returned to the previous, typical postmenopausal levels.

Since this initial, provocative research, the estrogenic potential of plant estrogens has been demonstrated repeatedly. In *Maturitas: Journal of Climacteric and Postmenopause*, A. L. Murikis reported an impressive reduction in menopausal symptoms from the ingestion of modest amounts of soy. Fifty-eight women whose average age was fifty-four and who had at least fourteen hot flashes a week supplemented their diets with about 45 grams (about 6 tablespoons) of soy flour a day. Within six weeks, they reported an average 40 percent reduction in menopausal discomforts, including hot flashes, sweats, palpitations, headaches, sleep disturbances, depression, tiredness, irritability/nervousness, frequent urge to urinate, vaginitis, and loss of libido.

In another study, reported in the *Journal of Endocrinology,* M. S. Morton found that flaxseed or soy elevated the levels of estrogen in blood plasma within two weeks. Postmenopausal women ate a diet supplemented with about 6 tablespoons of soy flour or 2 tablespoons of flaxseed daily. Consuming flaxseed resulted in particularly dramatic estrogenic increases.

These studies do not stand alone. Research demonstrating elevated levels of plant estrogen in the urine of women eating soy and flaxseed has been reported in the *Journal of the American Dietetic Association,* the *Journal of the Society for Experimental Biology and Medicine,* the *Journal of the American Society of Clinical Nutrition,* and *Cancer Epidemiology.*

Laboratory research has confirmed the estrogenic effects of soy and flaxseed. Neerja Sathymoorthy of the Cancer Research and Development Center has introduced a method for demonstrating the estrogenic responses of cells to different forms of estrogen. He compared the effects of pharmaceutical estrogen with the effects of plant estrogens. The plant estrogens in flaxseed and soy showed significant estrogenic activity.

In addition to research studies and laboratory experiments, cultural comparison suggests that foods rich in plant estrogens can both relieve menopausal distress and protect against breast cancer. In her book *The Estrogen Decision,* Susan Lark, M.D., reports the difference in incidence of menopausal symptoms in the United States and Japan. In the United States between 80 and 85 percent of women suffer menopausal symptoms of overheating and "drying up"—hot flashes, night sweats, vaginal dryness, dry skin, mood swings, irritability, depression, anxiety, tiredness, poor concentration, memory loss, loss of sexual desire, and urinary-tract problems. In Japan—where soy products, especially tofu, are a staple in a low-fat diet—only 10 to 15 percent of women experience these symptoms. Not only do women in America endure more discomfort during menopause, they have a higher incidence of breast cancer. According to statistics reported in *Cancer Facts and Figures,* a publication of the American Cancer Society, women in the United States are four and a half times more likely to die of breast cancer than women in Japan.

▧ SOY AND CANCER PROTECTION

The power of the soybean appears to contribute to the extraordinary disparity in breast cancer rates in the United States and Japan. Many studies comparing groups of people who regularly eat soy products and those who eat less or no soy point to its cancer-protective potential. With few exceptions, the epidemiological data indicate that eating whole, nonfermented soy products (especially tofu and soy milk) regularly predicts lower rates of breast cancer. Women are less likely to develop breast cancer if they eat tofu or soy milk once a day than if they eat tofu or soy milk twice a week. In a pioneering study reported in *Lancet,* H. P. Lee examined the diet of 620 women living in Singapore. Those who ate about two servings of soy per day were less than half as likely to develop breast cancer as those who seldom ate soy.

Serious laboratory research into the cancer-protective potential of soy began in 1989. Stephen Barnes, Ph.D., and Ken Setchell, Ph.D., added small amounts of soy to the diets of rats. The result was a 50 percent reduction in breast cancer. Other animal studies followed, indicating that soy reduced the risk of liver, bladder, stomach, prostate, and breast cancer.

Mark Messina, Ph.D., a former researcher at the National Cancer Institute, identifies seven components of soy that appear to offer protection from cancer:

1. *Protease inhibitors* in soy appear to interfere with the activation of genes associated with cancers of the colon, lung, pancreas, esophagus, and breast.
2. *Phytate* in soy acts like an antioxidant. It has been shown to impede both breast and colon cancer in laboratory experiments.
3. *Phytosterols* protect the colon from harmful bile acids. In addition to reducing colon tumors by 50 percent, phytosterols have been effective in reducing skin cancer in laboratory research.
4. *Saponins* are potentially cancer-protective antioxidants in soy. Under laboratory conditions, saponins have been shown to prevent mutations in cells that lead to cancer.
5. *Phenolic acid,* another antioxidant, appears to protect against mutations that lead to cancer.
6. *Lecithin* has reduced lung tumors in mice.
7. *Plant estrogens*—often referred to as *isoflavones* or *phytoestrogens*—have awakened the most excitement. Messina notes that while the other six components of soy are available in other foods, two particular plant estrogens—*genistein* and *daidzein*—are found almost exclusively in soy. Well over 750 papers investigating the cancer-protective potential of soy's estrogens have been published in medical journals.

Much of this soy-estrogen research has been undertaken in test tubes or petri dishes. It's the cheapest, quickest way to screen substances for their cancer-protective potential. When the soy estrogen genistein has been added to cancerous and normal cells, it inhibits the growth of the cancer cells but does not interfere with the growth of normal cells. Under laboratory conditions, genistein even causes cancer cells to revert back to normal cells.

Likewise, in animal research, soy's plant estrogens appear to account for much of soy's cancer-protective results. To follow up his previous research, Stephen Barnes fed whole soybean meal and soy with plant estrogens removed to animals that were genetically predisposed to breast cancer and that had been injected with breast cancer cells. The animals that received whole soy got 50 percent less cancer than the animals that ate soy without plant estrogens.

Recently, intriguing evidence was added to the ever-increasing case for soy as breast cancer protection. The American Society of Experimental Biology reported a study conducted by A. Cassidy. Soy was added to the diets of premenopausal women for two months. Two important changes occurred in these women: First, their menstrual cycles increased by about two and a half days. (A longer menstrual cycle is associated with a lower risk of breast cancer.) Second, the blood levels of estrogen-related pituitary hormones decreased substantially—a result similar to the effect of tamoxifen, a widely prescribed cancer-fighting drug. Tamoxifen neutralizes the cancer-promoting potential of the strong estrogens (estradiol and estrone). Researchers believe soy estrogens may work in the same way, having the same neutralizing effect.

▧ FLAXSEED AND BREAST CANCER PROTECTION

Flaxseed also appears to fight breast cancer. In seminars given to physicians, Jeffrey Bland, Ph.D., reports his own experience—how he unexpectedly pioneered investigation into the potentially breast cancer–protective benefits of flaxseed oil. While working at the Linus Pauling Institute, Bland and fellow researchers undertook a study of the effects of fat on breast cancer development in laboratory mice. They divided three hundred mice into six groups of fifty. All the mice had been bred to be at high risk for breast cancer. All were fed identical diets, but five of the six groups were given additional fat. One group ate corn oil, the second ate lard, the third ate flaxseed oil, the fourth ate fish oil, the fifth ate evening primrose oil, and the sixth, the control group, ate no supplemental fat. The five groups eating a diet supplemented with oil were also given a carcinogen. The control group received no carcinogen. The research was designed as a "blind" study—the researchers did not know which groups of animals were being fed which oils. After forty-two weeks, all fifty of the mice in four of the groups had died, while all fifty of the mice in two of the groups remained alive. Since the control group had received no additional carcinogen, Bland and his colleagues assumed one of the living groups would be the control group. To their surprise, all of the mice in the control group had died. The two groups that lived were fed a diet supplemented with flaxseed oil or fish oil—oils rich in omega-3 essential fatty acids. Research sponsored by the American Health Foundation found comparable results. Mice fed diets high in omega-3 fatty acids were 40 percent less likely to develop metastatic breast cancer than mice fed on corn oil. Demographic studies confirm that breast cancer is less prevalent when omega-3 oils have a prominent place in the diet.

Current research on the implications of flaxseed for breast cancer focuses on its plant estrogen content. Flaxseed is rich in plant estrogens called *lignans*. While researchers repeatedly find high concentrations of lignans in herbal remedies used in Chinese, Indian, Native American, Mexican, South American, Indonesian, and Korean traditional medicines, these potent substances are hard to find in food. At the University of Toronto, Lillian Thompson, Ph.D., examined sixty-eight foods, searching for those high in lignans. She found that flaxseed contains between 75 and 800 times more lignans than any of the other foods.

In December 1994, the *Journal of the National Cancer Institute* reported that experiments done in the 1980s suggest lignans might have anticarcinogenic effects. The *Journal* described a variety of investigative approaches that appear to confirm the earlier suspicion. At the University of Minnesota and the University of Helsinki, researchers found that lignans inhibited estrogen production from fatty tissue—the primary source of postmenopausal cancer-implicated estrogen (estrone). Herman Adlercreutz, M.D., at the University of Helsinki, found that Finnish women who did not eat flaxseed bread were more likely to contract breast cancer than those who ate the bread regularly.

A number of animal studies have also provided evidence that flaxseed consumption may inhibit the development of breast as well as prostate and colon cancers. *Nutrition and Cancer* reported that when M. Serraino fed female mice that had been exposed to a chemical carcinogen a diet of 5 percent flaxseed, cancerous growths were significantly reduced—by 66.7 percent when compared to predicted rates. Lillian Thompson, Ph.D., found that rats fed flaxseed showed a 50 percent reduction in carcinogen-induced colon tumors. Cancer-affected breast cells were likewise reduced in number. In addition, Dr. Thompson found that when rats with established tumors were fed flaxseed, their tumors decreased.

William Phipps examined the benefits of flaxseed in yet another way. His results were reported in the *Journal of Clinical Endocrinology and Metabolism.* Researchers monitored premenopausal women for seven menstrual cycles. For three consecutive menstrual cycles, the researchers supplemented their diets with 10 grams of flaxseed powder (about 1 tablespoon of flaxseed) per day. This small amount of flaxseed resulted in significant changes in the women's menstrual cycles: the length of their cycles increased; their ratio of progesterone to estradiol increased; they ovulated with every cycle. In total, these positive changes are thought to be predictive of a reduced risk of breast cancer.

So, a substantial body of responsible research suggests that plant estrogens—soy and flaxseed—reduce the risk of breast cancer. How do they do it?

No one knows for sure, but researchers generally subscribe to one consistent theory: The biochemical structure of the plant estrogens is similar to those of the estrogens produced by women's bodies. Plant estrogens, however, are much weaker than the cancer-implicated estrogens estradiol and estrone. Despite their weakness, plant estrogens appear to travel through the bloodstream to estrogen-receptor sites in breasts and sexual organs. When they reach these receptor sites, they seem to latch on and take up residence. While they appear to have beneficial estrogenic effects—diminishing menopausal symptoms and positively affecting menstruation—they do not seem to exert harmful carcinogenic effects. As long as plant estrogens reside in the estrogen-receptor sites, there doesn't appear to be room for the cancer-implicated estrogens to move in and wreak havoc.

Following this logic, women who take hormone replacement therapy may decrease their risk of breast cancer by eating more soy and flaxseed. If plant estrogens guard estrogen-receptor sites from invasion by estradiol and estrone, soy and flaxseed may help women escape breast cancer.

Andrew Weil, M.D., the best-selling author of *Spontaneous Healing*, dispenses well-researched, responsible information. He recommends that menopausal women eat soy products and flaxseed for their potentially cancer-preventive benefits.

Women at risk for breast cancer may be the most tempted to exchange hormone replacement pills for a diet rich in plant estrogens. But women concerned about other long-term risks—cardiovascular disease and osteoporosis—may be more hesitant. Hormone replacement therapy has convincing benefits. Women may well wonder, "Will munching my way through menopause on foods rich in plant estrogens really provide protection for my heart and bones?" The research is well worth considering.

▧ HEARTFELT EFFECTS

Soy and flaxseed—these potential guardians against cancer—appear to protect hearts as well. And women's hearts need protection. After the age of fifty-five, women are ten times more likely to have a heart attack than before menopause. Heart disease is the number one killer of women in the United States. While about 40,000 women die from breast cancer each year, 500,000 die from cardiovascular disease.

There is little doubt that soy can be beneficial to the heart. The "heartfelt" effects of soy became headline news in August 1995, when the *New England Journal of Medicine* reported the combined results of thirty-eight research studies. All of the studies compared two groups of people. Both groups ate essentially the same diet, except that one group ate more than 30 grams of soy per day—two to three servings. The other group ate no soy. Compared to the non-soy eaters, the average overall cholesterol level of the soy-fed groups was reduced by 9.3 percent. Their "bad" cholesterol (LDL) decreased by 12.9 percent, and their "good" cholesterol (HDL) increased by 2.4 percent. The sound bite on the nightly news said simply: "The more soy you eat, the more you'll lower your cholesterol."

The authors of the study point to plant estrogens as the most likely reason for the cholesterol-lowering effect of soy. In research studies in which two groups of monkeys ate the same amount of soy protein, plant estrogens appeared to be the primary factor accounting for significant cholesterol decreases. One group ate soy with the plant estrogens removed, and the other group ate whole soy meal. The soy diet without plant estrogens resulted in minimal cholesterol reduction. The whole soy feed, rich in plant estrogens, lowered cholesterol significantly.

In Italy, researchers also achieved dramatic cholesterol-lowering effects. Research conducted by A. Gaddi and reported in the *American Journal of Nutrition* found that patients with familial hypercholesterolemia, a genetic condition that results in dangerously high cholesterol, showed little improvement from a low-fat diet but dramatic improvement from a diet rich in soy. When animal protein was replaced by soy protein, their cholesterol levels dropped 26 percent.

Other components of soy appear to make a contribution to maintaining healthy hearts. Soluble soy fiber has demonstrated modest cholesterol-lowering effects. Administered in large quantities, lecithin has been shown to lower cholesterol. Saponins and phytosterols have likewise produced cholesterol-lowering benefits. And the oil in soy contains about 8 percent omega-3 essential fatty acids. Omega-3s have repeatedly been associated with heart health.

While soy offers modest amounts of omega-3 essential fatty acids, flaxseed contains five times as much as any other commonly available plant food. These fatty acids are "essential" for health and survival, but the human body is incapable of producing them; they must be obtained from food. While a healthy diet should be reasonably low in total fat—about 20 to 25 percent—the fat we do eat should be rich in essential fatty acids—especially omega-3s. These healthy oils appear to relax our blood vessels, improve our circulation, protect our blood from unhealthy clotting, lower our blood pressure, and reduce inflammatory changes. Unlike the saturated fats in meat, milk, margarine, and coconut and palm oils, which increase cholesterol, flaxseed oil appears to lower cholesterol. So not only is flaxseed the richest known food source for plant estrogens, it's brimming with heart-healthy oil as well.

Flaxseed as well as flaxseed oil appears to enhance heart health. In the *British Medical Journal,* S. C. Cunnane described the effects of flaxseed on cholesterol. The diets of healthy young women (average age twenty-four) were supplemented with 50 grams of flaxseed flour (about 4 tablespoons of flaxseed) per day. After four weeks, their total cholesterol level was lowered by 9 percent. But more important, their LDL ("bad") cholesterol was lowered by 18 percent. The ratio of "good" to "bad" cholesterol was thus substantially improved. Comparable benefits were obtained when the flaxseed was consumed in muffins.

In a study of elderly people, published in the *Journal of the American College of Nutrition,* M. L. Bierenbaum reported similar effects. All of the participants in this study had been taking 800 I.U.s of vitamin E for a prolonged period. When 15 grams of ground flaxseed (about 4 teaspoons) and three slices of flaxseed bread were added to their diets, their total and their LDL cholesterol levels decreased significantly. Their HDL cholesterol level remained the same. Again, the ratio of "good" to "bad" cholesterol improved.

Alongside heart disease, osteoporosis is the other major debilitating danger that estrogen appears to prevent. Osteoporosis, from the Greek, literally means "porous bones." As women age, they face the risk of gradually losing bone mass. There is a very good chance that vast numbers of female baby boomers are going to grow old—very old. In *New Passages,* Gail Sheehy reports that women who reach age fifty without contracting heart disease or cancer can expect to live to be ninety-two. That's a lot of time for bones to bear. By age seventy-five, fully 45 percent of American women will suffer from extreme bone deterioration.

Losing estrogen and progesterone threatens the reserves of calcium in bones. Hormone replacement therapy appears to benefit bones. Estrogen seems to preserve bones, and progesterone actually seems to rebuild them. As long as women take hormone replacement therapy, their bones appear to be protected. As soon as they stop, deterioration resumes. That's why many doctors think that women who are at high risk for osteoporosis—those who are small-boned, fair-skinned, and blue-eyed—should take hormone replacement therapy forever. Even though the risk of breast cancer appears to mount the longer hormone replacement therapy is taken, the bone-preserving evidence in favor of hormone replacement therapy is strong—a fact not to be dismissed lightly.

For women troubled by the long-term effects of prolonged medication, it is reassuring to know that soy does appear to possess some bone-protective potential. Bone preservation requires a balance between calcium consumed and calcium excreted. To maintain bone mass, the body must take in at least as much calcium as it eliminates. In a study reported in the *Journal of Clinical Endocrinology and Metabolism,* Neil Breslau has compared how different types of protein affect calcium balance. All participants in his study ate the same amount of protein. One group ate meat and dairy; another ate soy. The group that ate meat and dairy lost 50 percent more calcium from their bodies than those who ate soy. Studies consistently show that those who rely on soy rather than meat excrete less urinary calcium.

Animal research has also confirmed the bone-beneficial value of soy. In a study reported in *Endocrinology,* Dike Kalu examined the bone health of rats fed on soy protein compared to milk protein. Rats fed soy experienced delayed onset of bone loss and lost significantly less bone. The author suggested that eating soy at an early age may prevent osteoporosis.

Among soy-protein products, tofu is particularly beneficial to women concerned about the continued strength of their bones. Tofu is an excellent source of calcium. While a glass of milk offers about 325 mg of calcium, a quarter of a cake (4 ounces) of firm tofu made with calcium sulfate provides about 550 mg. Calcium, like all minerals and unlike vitamins, is not damaged when cooked.

In addition to soy's seemingly bone-beneficial protein and calcium, its plant estrogens may also contribute to bone strength. In their exhaustive review of the scientific literature, *The Simple Soybean and Your Health,* researchers Mark Messina, Virginia Messina, and Ken Setchell report an intriguing development. Ipriflavone is a drug widely used in Italy and Japan as an accepted preventive and treatment for bone loss. The name *Ipriflavone* closely resembles the word *isoflavone*—a commonly used name for soy plant estrogens. The similarity in the two names is not a coincidence. The chemical structure of Ipriflavone and of soy estrogens resemble one another. In the body, one of the breakdown products of Ipriflavone is actually daidzein—one of the major plant estrogens found naturally in soy. While systematic studies have yet to be conducted on the bone-protective effects of daidzein, its biochemical similarity to Ipriflavone suggests it may have bone-protective potential.

Women at high risk for osteoporosis need to attend to their bones. Along with a carefully considered decision about the benefits and risks of hormone replacement therapy versus a diet rich in soy and flaxseed, long-term bone health requires a commitment to lifestyle changes. Weight-bearing exercise and a diet rich in calcium and boron, along with vitamin and mineral supplements, are highly recommended. To protect their bones, women need to walk for one hour or train with weights for forty-five minutes at least three times a week. In addition, vitamin supplementation—calcium citrate plus the synergetic nutrients magnesium, boron, manganese, zinc, copper, and vitamin K—is highly beneficial.

☰ THE QUESTION OF QUANTITIES

G. B. Milis, in *Bone and Mineral,* advocates 6.25 mg of pharmaceutical estrogen to protect bone, but recent studies suggest that less may be sufficient. Researchers Morris Notelovitz and Karen Preswood found that 0.3 mg increased bone density and protected against bone loss. Given the relative weakness of plant estrogens compared to pharmaceutical estrogen, a question looms: Is it possible to get enough estrogenic effect from soy and flaxseed not only to relieve menopausal symptoms, reduce cancer risk, and lower cholesterol, but also to protect bones?

Surprisingly, reducing cancer risk and menopausal symptoms appears to require the smallest portion of daily soy intake. Researchers at Tufts University, the University of Alabama, the University of Helsinki, and the National Cancer Institute all report that ingesting one to two servings of soy per day appears to decrease breast cancer risk. Published studies in the *British Medical Journal* and *Maturitas* have demonstrated decreased menopausal symptoms in women eating the equivalent of one serving of soy per day. According to analyses reported in the *New England Journal of Medicine,* lowering cholesterol may require more soy—between two and three servings per day. As for protection from osteoporosis, the quantities appear to be considerable.

In the *Journal of the National Cancer Institute,* Mark Messina and Stephen Barnes report that 200 mg of soy plant estrogens equal .3 mg of pharmaceutical estrogen. Given their estimates, it would take about 420 mg of soy estrogens to approximate a bone-protective dose. At the 1990 National Cancer Institute–sponsored conference on the role of soy products in cancer prevention, Donna Baird reported that one main dish (½ cup of soybeans or 38 grams of texturized vegetable protein) plus two snacks (soy nuts or roasted soybean spread on crackers) equal about 200 mg of plant estrogen. Given these estimates, approximating a bone-protective dose would require between three and eight servings of soy per day. Nutritionally oriented physicians consider fewer portions of soy bone protective when combined with weight-bearing exercise and a diet rich in bone-protective minerals and vitamins, and vitamin and mineral supplements.

Determining the amount of flaxseed needed to approximate chemical estrogen requires careful consideration and more speculation. However, flaxseed does appear to contain a greater concentration of plant estrogens than soy. In multiple medical studies, smaller amounts of flaxseed result in similar estrogenic benefits. In a paper published in the *Proceedings of the Society for Experimental Biology and Medicine,* W. R. Obermeyer of the Food and Drug Administration identified flaxseed as "potentially the richest source" of plant estrogens. One tablespoon of flaxseed appears to be roughly comparable to one serving of soy. Considering all current research reviewed, 1 tablespoon of flaxseed may reduce breast cancer risk, 2 tablespoons appears to diminish menopausal discomfort, and 3 to 5 tablespoons seems to lower cholesterol. No research examining the bone-protective potential of flaxseed has been reviewed. However, if plant estrogens offer safeguards similar to those of pharmaceutical estrogen, 3 to 8 tablespoons of flaxseed might offer a bone-protective dose. Some nutritionally focused physicians suggest the smaller amounts of flaxseed may reduce osteoporosis risk when combined with weight-bearing exercise, a diet rich in bone-protective minerals and vitamins, and vitamin and mineral supplements.

⧼ FLAXSEED AND SOY: BENEFITS FOR EVERY WOMAN

For all our investigation, we can't be absolutely sure that soy and flaxseed will safeguard women's breasts, hearts, and bones for the long term. Nor do we know if the benefits of hormone replacement therapy are worth the risk.

All authorities agree on one conclusion: We won't know for ten years whether the risks of combined conventional hormone replacement therapy are greater than the benefits. How will we know? The calculations will be made. We'll tabulate how many women have gotten breast cancer, how many have died from heart disease, and how many have broken bones. We will know when, and only when, some of our friends, partners, and patients have become statistics.

In the meantime, whatever your choice about hormone replacement therapy, it can't hurt to take good care of yourself—to eat more consciously and exercise more regularly. No matter what your decision, foods rich in plant estrogen—soy and flaxseed—appear to offer increased safety. Eating soy and flaxseed as an integrated part of a balanced, whole-food, calcium- and mineral-rich diet appears to add an extra measure of protection from all these risks without increasing any of them. By incorporating soy and flaxseed into their diets, women who take hormone replacement therapy may add an extra measure of protection against any possible increased risk of breast cancer.

As for those who cannot tolerate the side effects or bear the insecurities that come with hormone replacement therapy, consciously caring for themselves requires taking an "alternative" path. We know many women plagued by side effects from estrogen and progesterone. Most often they report unrelenting nausea or perpetual PMS. While these symptoms can be modified by lowering doses or using alternative hormone replacement therapy, many physicians and women remain uncomfortable with this option. The June 26, 1995, issue of *Time* magazine reported that estrogen had already become the most prescribed drug in America. In that same article, Claudia Wallace cited a 1987 survey that reported that 20 percent of women who get a prescription for hormone replacement therapy have second thoughts on their way to the drugstore—and never fill the prescription. Of those who begin taking hormone replacement therapy, one third stop within nine months, and half quit by the end of a year. The magazine estimated that three out of four women between forty-five and sixty-four do not take hormone replacement therapy. For these women, a paper published in the May 1996 issue of *Obstetrics & Gynecology* may offer encouragement. Knight and Eden reviewed 861 relevant articles from reputable medical journals and concluded that estrogen-rich foods, particularly soy and flaxseed, may offer "a safe, cheap, generally side effect–free alternative to current pharmaceutical measures (HRT).

This decision to forgo medical intervention does not set minds at ease. Women wonder and worry. To feel confident, they need to consider alternatives to hormone replacement therapy—to find other ways to replenish dwindling supplies of vital hormones. An estrogen-packed diet has been shown to help. Eating foods that restore estrogen may bring some relief. Of course, any foods, including soy and flaxseed, may cause allergic reactions in a small number of people. And all women who are taking any medication, including hormone replacement therapy, should consult with their physician when they are considering making any major dietary changes. But diet is only one part of living a health-promoting life. Exercise, Chinese medicine, Western herbs, homeopathic remedies, vitamin supplements, and other natural hormonal products deserve investigation. In this stage of a woman's life, if she doesn't pay attention to her needs, her body will force her to pay attention to its deterioration. Menopause is a time to nurture yourself—to care and cook for yourself.

ESTROGEN: THE NATURAL WAY

One

Searching for Safe Passage: My Story

Estrogen makes me sick. Really. Literally.

Here I am. A menopausal woman. Blond, blue-eyed, small-boned. A picture of osteoporosis waiting to happen. Soaking in my own sweat. Waking up at two-hour intervals every single night by a self-generated tropical typhoon. With each awakening, I feel the force of realization: "I'm burning up. I'm drying out. *I'm becoming a prune!* Soon, I'll be old, frail, haggard. *I'm at risk.* I need help."

So I go to my doctor. He looks at me, raises all-knowing eyebrows, and says, "You need to take hormone replacement therapy." I ask, "Will the sheets stay dry?" He answers, "Yes, and your bones will stay strong, your heart will stay healthy, your skin will stay young and . . . you'll maintain vaginal lubrication." I consider his predictions. He's telling me I'll sleep without sweat in a revitalized, vibrant, sexy body. So what's not to like? I ask, "What about breast cancer?" He says, "You're not at high risk for breast cancer." I say, "I know." I think to myself, "Neither are most of the one in eight women who get it." I repress the thought. I behave like a good patient. I'm grateful. I take the prescription. I clutch it in my clammy palm.

I go directly to the drugstore—mobilized by hope, confident that the medicine will soothe my sweltering body and forestall the ravages of aging. I get my pills—little miracle potions. I gobble them up. I wait.

The day after my first dose, I woke up nauseous. The next day, I woke up with nausea and a headache. I felt pregnant. The first three months of each of my pregnancies had been the worst times of my entire life, but at least I had gotten two babies out of it. What was I going to get out of this? Strong bones, healthy teeth, and perpetual PMS? I started eating saltines, guzzling ginger ale, and taking vitamin B_6. I got no relief. I came to a paranoid epiphany: Hormone replacement therapy is a male conspiracy designed to keep women subservient—just sick and insecure enough to function with minimal competence; able to make beds and vacuum floors but incapable of writing financial reports and running board meetings. I blamed the nearest representative of the dominant gender: I grumped at my husband, Michael. He tiptoed around, hoping to keep a safe distance. I glared when he passed through my field of vision. He looked for a reason for my scornful scowls. I assured him, "It's not personal. It's not your fault you're a *man.*"

Two weeks went by. I continued stuffing my face with saltines every morning, afternoon, and evening. I bought gallons of ginger ale to wash down the buffered aspirin I popped three or four at a time. Out of empathy for my mate, I made a decision. I instructed myself: "Don't trust anything you think. If you believe your mind, you'll attack. It'll be ugly." I tried to contain my seething hormones. They built. They swelled. Finally, I burst in rebellion. I made a rash and inadvisable decision. Instead of gradually decreasing my dosage as responsible physicians recommend, I threw the estrogen and the progesterone into the wastebasket. I announced, "No man is going to do this to me." I told my husband, "You're just going to have to accept it. I'm growing old gracefully." He assured me, "That's fine, honey. I liked you better before you took the hormones."

Two days later the sheets were wet when I turned over. I looked at the man I've loved for twenty-five years and felt grateful for the time we'd weathered together. I reached out to hold his hand. His eyes opened. He saw my gaze. He sighed, "That's better."

But recovering my emotional security didn't secure me a good night's sleep. I needed some relief. I still felt like a middle-aged bed wetter. I had no control. Like clockwork every two hours—at 11 P.M., at 1 A.M., at 3 A.M., at 5 A.M., and at 7 A.M.—perspiration streamed out of every pore of my body. I woke up boiling and threw the covers off. For maybe three minutes, I felt comfortably warm. Then, my drenched nightshirt turned cold. Now I was swaddled in chilled, dampened, absorbent cotton. I pulled the covers back over me. My moist cotton nightclothes gradually warmed. I returned to sleep for another hour and a half before my temperature rose once again.

For the first time in my life, I wondered how my mother had endured menopause. I only vaguely recalled her menopause. I had been a teenager, with teachers, friends, and boys to impress; my mom's menopausal woes had made no impression on me. Thirty-five years later, I was finally interested. I sat down with her to talk. I asked, "Was menopause difficult for you?" She looked at me in disbelief. "Don't you remember? I had five D and Cs. I went to the hospital every other year for ten years." I confessed, "I remember we used to tease you about your biannual trips to the hospital, but I didn't remember they were because of menopause." I asked her how long she had taken estrogen. She thought for a moment, then said, "For a long time. I don't remember exactly. At least ten years. Probably fifteen." I said, "That's probably why you had to have all those D and Cs." She responded, "Maybe. But without the estrogen, my hot flashes would have been much worse." I was surprised by this news. "You still had hot flashes even when you took estrogen?" She laughed and said, "I had lots of hot flashes. I still have hot flashes." That last bit of information seemed unbelievable. "Mom, you're over seventy-five." She corrected me, "I'm seventy-nine." My sprightly little mom was nearly eighty and she was still going through menopause! I was amazed. She played it down: "I only have them a few times a week. Your grandmother had them much worse. They never stopped. She had them her whole life." I assessed my situation. I thought, "It's hereditary. I'd better accept my fate. From now until I am very, very old, I can expect sudden-onset sweats."

Not long after my meeting with my mom, my friend Martin Bock, an acupuncturist and Chinese herbalist, called. He asked about my discomfort and made an offer: "Would you like me to send you some herbs?" I answered, "Please. Thank you." I was willing to try anything. Secretly, I feared my desperation had gotten me into boiling foul-smelling brews like the ones my husband ingested during allergy season. A few days later a package arrived. Martin had sent me powder and drops. I was relieved. I began taking the herbs. Within a week my ten-minute night sweats turned into five-minute heat waves. Instead of being visited upon me every two hours, they came at three-hour intervals. I dropped in and out of sleep more restfully.

Back in balance, I started searching for alternatives to hormone replacement therapy—other ways to protect my bones, heart, and breasts. Right on cue, as though written especially to me, the front page of *The Boston Globe* announced: "Inside this edition you will find directions for navigating the maze of the estrogen replacement debate." Reporter Judy Forman informed me that pumping iron might be just as effective as estrogen for protecting my pitifully petite skeleton. I vowed to continue jumping on our weight-training machine every other day. I read on. She advised making sure to get enough calcium: "Eat your green vegetables and drink your milk." No problem. I drank a quart of chocolate skim milk a day plus a cup or two of decaf latte. I liked this lady. She was telling me what I wanted to hear. I continued reading. Then, suddenly—without warning—she sprang this bad news on me. She said soybeans had estrogen and that Japanese women—who eat lots of tofu—had fewer menopausal symptoms than American women. I hated tofu. I quickly decided, "I'm at low risk for heart disease and for breast cancer. I'll trust the long-term benefits of exercise and milk. Forget the tofu."

But the media refused to leave me in peace. Gail Sheehy's *New Passages* hit number one on *The New York Times* best-seller list. My husband bought it. He read me bedtime stories about the wonders of estrogen: "Estrogen Makes You Sexy," "Estrogen Makes You Strong." I turned over. "I know those stories. I'm not impressed. I'm making lifestyle changes. I'm working out, eating well, taking Chinese herbs. I'll be sexy and strong."

Just when I thought I was safe, he read me a new story: "Estrogen Makes You Smart." "Listen to this," he reported. " 'Women who take estrogen are less likely to suffer from Alzheimer's disease and score better on memory tests.' " At that point, he got my attention. I cared about smart. I didn't want to grow into an old, oversexed female hulk without a brain. I confessed what I knew. "I read that tofu contains estrogen naturally. Japanese women have fewer symptoms during menopause." Worried, I wondered out loud, "Do you think tofu protects their minds?" Thinking quickly, he tried to console me. "Men in Japan eat tofu too. Maybe it protects everybody's intelligence—both men and women." He was trying very hard to be sweet. "But what," I asked myself, "is this perfectly intelligent man trying to tell me now? That if the entire American auto industry ate massive quantities of tofu, they'd make better cars and solve the trade deficit?"

≋ EXPLORING THE POWER OF PLANT ESTROGENS

The next day I woke up thinking, "I've got to find out about tofu. I need to know if this soy-estrogen connection is for real."

Off I trotted to the book section of our natural foods supermarket. I piled thirteen books with *menopause* or *estrogen* in their titles into my shopping cart. I settled in for days, reading up on all the latest. Next, I left the world of natural nutritional alternatives and went in search of more sources. I planted myself in the reading corners of every academic and mainstream bookstore within a twenty-mile radius of my home.

I discovered that tofu is not the only food rich in plant estrogens. Every soy product ever produced—soybeans, soy nuts, soy milk, texturized vegetable protein, plus some of those fake sausages and hamburgers—contains plant estrogen. And then there was flaxseed. What was it? All I knew was that it was an edible seed of some kind. I figured I'd find out more about flaxseed later. Right then, all I wanted to know was, "Can I really get estrogen without getting sick?"

As I read, I learned the scientific code name for all plant estrogen: *phytoestrogen*. As soon as this word popped up, the article writers—physicians and nutritionists—started talking about breast cancer protection. Suddenly, I was confused. I thought estrogen *increased* breast cancer risk. But right in front of me, in black and white, expert after expert was saying that plant estrogens might *reduce* breast cancer risk. I was skeptical. Could this really be true?

I put together bits and pieces of information. It turned out I'd been deluded. I had thought there was one estrogen. It turns out that there are many different forms of estrogen, all with different names. Biochemically speaking, they look alike, but they have different strengths and different names. Three—estradiol, estrone, and estriol—are produced in our bodies—yours and mine. I tried to understand without getting overwhelmed. Estradiol and estrone are strong estrogens. Estriol is a weak estrogen. Plant estrogens—which come in many varieties—are also weak estrogens.

In healthy numbers and for a limited amount of time, strong estrogens circulate through our systems, doing beneficial work—keeping our bones strong, our hearts healthy, our skin wrinkle-free, our sexual juices flowing. But if too many strong estrogens circulate through our systems for too long, they can turn on us. Strong estrogens tend to befriend breast cancer. Maybe they cause the cancer. Maybe they just activate the cancer. But they certainly become cancer's ally, supporting the disease as it wages war on our bodies.

While an overabundance of strong estrogens places us in harm's way, weak estrogens may offer some protection from their more toxic family members. These weak estrogens appear to latch on to estrogen-receptor sites in our breasts and uterus. Once they latch on, they seem to stand guard, making it more difficult for the potentially destructive estrogens to get in and wreak havoc.

How do we get too much strong estrogen? It seems a mystery, really, but there are clues. When we menstruate longer—in other words, start early and stop late—our bodies manufacture more strong estrogens. When we are overweight, our fat cells produce more strong estrogens. Both put us at greater risk for breast cancer. And here's the scary part.

When we take conventional estrogen replacement therapy, we pop the strong estrogens—estradiol and estrone—in pill form. Premarin is estradiol—the strongest estrogen—synthesized from mare's urine. Just when our bodies are saying, "I don't feel like making strong estrogen anymore," we pump ourselves full of the most potent of estrogens.

Just as I was ready to get sanctimonious, I told myself, "Don't go off on some conspiracy theory about the pharmaceutical industry trying to keep women sexy and kill us simultaneously. Do we have choices? What happens without estrogen? For many of us it might just be a feverish downhill slide toward the ravages of old age—a sexless journey toward heart disease, osteoporosis, and dementia. Who wants to go on that ride willingly?"

Premarin may come with its own perils, but for many of us it works. For some of us it slows the inevitable and makes the journey more comfortable. If it didn't make me sick, I'd be taking it. But I'd be scared. I'd be nervous about breast cancer.

Enough about those strong estrogens with their ugly underside. What about weak estrogens? Were they really dependably benevolent? Could they be trusted to ward off their overpotent siblings?

Having exhausted all the available literature, I drove to the nearest medical school library. I wasn't ready to entrust my aging to a spattering of information. I wanted to read the original research myself. I wanted to make sure those health-crazed types weren't exaggerating or misleading the gullible among us.

I planted myself in front of a computer screen that read "*Welcome to OVID.*" This territory was new for me. I needed a guide. A research librarian patiently taught me how to access the database. I typed in one word—*soy*—and the computer screen flashed "656 citations." *OVID* could show me abstracts of 656 recent medical journal articles that had examined soy. I plugged in another word: *flaxseed. OVID* had fifty-seven abstracts in its files. With this resource at my fingertips, I became an information-age addict—a menopausal woman on a personal mission.

I traveled back to the medical library day after day. I stared at the computer screen. Often the abstracts were too technical for me to decipher.

But even the most daunting articles in the most scientific of journals—the *New England Journal of Medicine,* the *British Medical Journal,* the *Journal of Steroid Biochemistry,* and the *Journal of Clinical Endocrinology and Metabolism*—frequently worded their conclusions in understandable English. Bleary-eyed but obsessed, I read on, and on, and on. I printed every abstract I could comprehend about soy-plant estrogens. I printed all fifty-seven articles on flaxseed. Not content with abstracts, I searched the bookshelves. I copied entire articles. At home, I studied them with a medical dictionary in hand. Most of the articles focused on the potentially cancer-protective benefits of soy and flaxseed. I organized these into stacks of studies. I made notes about breast cancer research:

STACKS OF STUDIES

Stack 1—Epidemiological Studies: compare people's eating habits
　　Results: Women who eat lots of plant estrogens suffer from less breast cancer than women who don't eat lots of plant estrogens.

Stack 2—Animal Studies: compare rats
　　Results: When animals are exposed to carcinogens, the animals fed plant estrogens (soy or flaxseed) have fewer, smaller tumors than the animals who are not fed plant estrogens (soy or flaxseed).

Stack 3—Laboratory Studies: watch what happens to cells in petri dishes
　　Results: When cell tissue is exposed to carcinogens, the tissue also exposed to plant estrogens is less likely to become cancerous than the tissue not exposed to plant estrogens.

Stack 4—Human Studies: watch what happens to people under controlled conditions
　　Results: When premenopausal women supplement their usual diets with plant estrogens (soy or flaxseed), their hormones change in ways that reduce their risk for breast cancer.

These studies of soy and flaxseed don't deal solely with their potential for decreasing breast cancer. They also look at their effects on menopausal symptoms, cholesterol, and bones. All tend toward the positive: positive for diminishing menopausal symptoms; positive for lowering cholesterol; positive for benefiting bones.

I was impressed. I asked myself, "Should I begin my own plant-estrogen trial? Should I make myself into a menopausal pioneer—a soy/flaxseed guinea pig?"

Before I set out on that journey, I had to count calories.

▩ ESSENTIAL OILS: NATURE'S MOISTURE

Gone were the days when I was too thin. I looked back nostalgically to the time when I was constitutionally unable to gain weight. There had been a time when I could eat a bagel with a quarter pound of cream cheese every morning and chocolate mousse every night and never weigh more than ninety-six pounds. Not any longer. Two weeks after I turned forty-seven I had my first hot flash. Two days later, I stood in front of the mirror, nude. It was undeniable. I saw it—indisputable evidence of middle age—a potbellied protrusion on my own body. I looked four months pregnant. In tears, I dissolved into Michael's arms. I knew the truth. I had to stop eating cream. That day, I swore off high-calorie food and took up weight training.

Hard work and disciplined eating had kept my little protruding tummy in check. I didn't want the bulge back. The vanity police paraded through my mind screaming, "Are you nuts? Have you checked the calorie count of all this soy and flax stuff? What's the fat content? Who do you think you are? Do you think you can eat elephant-size portions of fatty food and not gain weight? Those days are gone, baby. Remember, you're a menopausal women. You gain two pounds when you look at a chocolate sundae. The omega-3 oils in flaxseed and soybeans may be good for your heart, but what will they do to your waistline?"

I decided to do some charting. I made a list of soy foods and flaxseed, including protein, calories, percentage of calories from fat, and grams of fat. I made another list of comparable conventional foods.

Comparing the totals, I found that on the whole, an estrogenic diet would give me more protein with fewer calories and less than

PLANT ESTROGEN FOOD	SERVING SIZE	PROTEIN GRAMS	CALORIES	% FAT CALORIES	FAT GRAMS
Soy Milks					
Silk	1 cup	4	80	25%	2.5
Soy Moo (fat free)	1 cup	7	110	0%	0
Soy West "Plus"	1 cup	6	150	32%	5
Soy Flour	½ cup	23.5	165	3%	0.5
Soy Nuts	½ cup	34	387	40%	18.6
Tofu					
Silken (Nasoya)	4¾ ounces	7.5	75	40%	3
Firm	4 ounces	12.8	118	54%	7.1
Mori-Nu (Low fat)	6 ounces	12	70	28%	2
Soft	4 ounces	9.4	88	57%	5.6
Soy "Meats"					
Boca Burger	1 burger	12	84	0%	0
Smart Dogs	1 link	9	45	0%	0
Gimme Lean	4 ounces	18	140	0%	0
Italian Links	1 link	5	60	30%	18
Flaxseed	3 tablespoons	5	140	64%	10
TOTALS		**165.2**	**1712**	**26%** (average)	**72.4**

CONVENTIONAL FOOD	SERVING SIZE	PROTEIN GRAMS	CALORIES	% FAT CALORIES	FAT GRAMS
Milks					
1 percent	1 cup	8	102	23%	2.6
Fat-free	1 cup	8	80	0%	0
Whole	1 cup	8	150	49%	8
Wheat Flour	½ cup	8.2	203	5%	1.1
Peanuts	½ cup	20.6	426	71%	36
Dairy Products					
Sour cream	¼ cup	2	110	85%	10
Cottage cheese	4 ounces	14.1	117	40%	5.1
Ricotta cheese	4 ounces	12	200	65%	15
Eggs	2	12.4	144	62%	10
Meat					
Burger	3 ounces	19.6	244	67%	17.8
Frankfurter	1 link	5.8	149	82%	14
Ground beef	4 ounces	18	350	78%	30
Sausage	1 link	3	130	87%	12
Sesame Seeds	3 tablespoons	6.3	141	77%	13.2
Totals		**146**	**2546**	**56.5%** (average)	**174.8**

half the fat of "conventional" foods. Some individual plant estrogen–rich foods are higher in fat than their common counterparts, but most are lower. Some, particularly the meat-mimicking products, are much lower. By using these foods in combination, it would be easy to keep my total fat intake between 20 and 30 percent—the level recommended by most cautious nutritionists and physicians. Since a high-fat diet does place women at greater risk for breast cancer as well as heart disease, it's important to keep one's diet within these boundaries.

Of course, the fat in plant estrogen–rich foods is a much healthier form of fat than that found in conventional foods. Almost none of it is saturated. None contains cholesterol. Nearly all of the oil in highly estrogenic food comes from essential fatty acids, with a large dose of potentially heart-saving, cholesterol-lowering omega-3s. Personally, I didn't need to worry about a super-low-fat, heart-disease-reversing diet. My cholesterol was low—about 150. My blood pressure was also low—about 125 over 68.

To maintain an estrogenic diet *and* maintain my weight, I'd need to be conscientious. I'd have to stay away from eggs, whole-fat dairy products, conventional baked goods, oil, nuts, meat, and—the only real sacrifice—chocolate bars. I'd need to make certain to balance my diet with lots of fruits, vegetables, and grains. I wouldn't be able to just add plant-estrogen foods to my diet; they'd have to *replace* other foods in my diet. I'd have to start getting more of my nutritional needs met from soy and flaxseed. Since soy is a protein-rich food packed with vitamins and minerals, and flaxseed contains healthful quantities of protein, minerals, and vitamins, that wasn't a problem.

Just as I was considering the fat in my menopausal diet, *The Zone* hit the best-seller list. Barry Sears and Bill Lawren asserted that fat was okay if kept in proper balance with proteins and carbohydrates. They also said that tofu had an excellent balance. They even called it a "protein-rich low-fat choice." I was beginning to feel reassured.

I took out another book I had learned to trust—*Menopause Without Medicine.* In it Linda Ojeda, Ph.D., cautions against a diet too low in fat. She voices concern that in our enthusiasm for cutting out fat, we will deprive ourselves of essential fatty acids. She points out that essential fatty acids—particularly omega-3s—moisturize the skin, the hair, and the genital tissue. By excluding these oils from our diet, we may increase vaginal dryness and promote premature wrinkles. Estrogen is only one factor in keeping the skin vital and the vaginal lining supple; we also need essential oils. Flaxseed and soybeans combined have more plant estrogen and essential fatty acids than any other vegetable foods.

I didn't want to shrivel up. I looked around. I saw the flaming fifties evaporating moisture out of skin. I compared women in their late forties and late fifties. By sixty sag sets in and wrinkles reign. I was entering the decade of deterioration—the time when people stop saying, "You look good" and start saying, "You look good *for your age.*"

Nor was I ready for my sexual juices to vaporize. With Manju living in New York and Sara nearly ready for college, Michael and I looked forward to reigniting our romance. I didn't want the time of hot flashes to dampen the heat of passion.

If soybeans and flaxseed could help to keep my skin vibrant and my sex life lively, I could handle counting the calories a little more carefully.

≋ MY PLANT ESTROGEN DECISION

Before deciding to embark on my own soybean-and-flaxseed trial run, I added up the pluses and the minuses.

POTENTIAL PLANT ESTROGEN POSITIVES	PLANT ESTROGEN NEGATIVES
• Minimize menopausal discomforts • Lower cholesterol • Benefit bones • Reduce risk of breast cancer • Maintain younger-looking skin • Maintain vaginal moisture	• Need to minimize conventional fat-rich foods

The potential outweighed the risk. I was convinced, but I still had to consider a basic question: "How much do I need to eat?"

〰 HOW MUCH PLANT ESTROGEN?

To figure out how much soy and flaxseed might stave off disease and deterioration, I pulled all my books, articles, and abstracts off the shelves. Nearly every human experiment fed women flaxseed or soy flour. They take a sort of "daily dose" approach, but there is no single minimum daily requirement for every benefit. Instead, there appears to be four different potentially effective doses: one to reduce the risk of breast cancer, another to diminish menopausal symptoms, a third to lower cholesterol, and a fourth to benefit bones.

Judging from the research, one serving of soy a day may reduce the risk of breast cancer; one to two servings may diminish menopausal symptoms; and two to five servings may lower cholesterol. The research on flaxseed is not as extensive, but there are promising indications that the same benefits may be available from flaxseed in small doses: 1 tablespoon may reduce the risk of breast cancer; 2 to 3 tablespoons may diminish menopausal symptoms; and 2 to 5 tablespoons may lower cholesterol.

Plant estrogens looked like good preventive medicine, but I was just coming to my own bone-breaking challenge—osteoporosis. Here's where my pitifully petite frame needed some support. It's not a pretty picture, this disease that secretly eats away at the skeleton. Osteoporosis slowly feeds on bones, filling them with tiny holes, infiltrating them with empty pockets. Like a termite-ridden house, the frame of a women with osteoporosis can't support her structure. Women with osteoporosis look and feel old. Shrunken. Hunched over. Humpbacked. Their stomachs stick out. They walk with a slow shuffle, afraid of falling and ashamed of their appearance. Personally, that portrait petrified me.

The osteoporosis threat—that's what my careful, conscientious, conservative, conventional doctor wanted to protect me from. That's really why he was so eager to write me a prescription for hormone replacement therapy. He wanted me to start taking those pills and continue to refill the prescription until the day I died.

Could plant estrogens really bolster my bones? Probably, if I ate enough of them. According to research estimates, it takes three to eight servings of soy a day or 3 to 8 tablespoons of flaxseed a day to approach an approximation of a bone-protective dose of estrogen.

≋ THE NEVER-ENDING DECISION

Still, to eat six to eight servings of soy or flaxseed daily meant a major commitment. I decided to make the commitment. I wasn't deceiving myself. I knew I was making up my own experiment in menopausal self-care. But hormone replacement therapy made me feel awful, and I was scared by the possibility of increasing my breast cancer risk, even a little.

Just as I was committing myself to a life of plant estrogen eating, in walked Melly. I met Melly in college. She was two years older than I, and I adored her. Admiration turned into long-lasting friendship. After we hugged, Melly confessed, "I'm taking hormone replacement therapy. My cholesterol is just too high. And I'm losing bone mass fast. I decided to break down and do it."

I felt relieved. Melly's mom died much too young. I didn't want to lose Melly. I worried about her health. I said, "I'm so glad."

Melly's decision made me wonder, "Will I be able to avoid hormone replacement therapy for the rest of my life? Will the danger to my bones become too great? Will I be able to forgo the medically prescribed solution?" I decided to do what was best for me one step at a time—to take vitamins, to do weight-bearing exercise, to drink Chinese herbs, and to eat soy and flaxseed—all the while keeping tabs on my bone density and getting my annual mammograms. I decided not to make any absolute, unchangeable decisions.

Melly and I sat down to talk. I told her about an interview I had heard on National Public Radio with Susan Love, M.D., who wrote *Dr. Susan Love's Breast Book*. I recalled her saying that many researchers now think latent breast cancer lives in every woman. In some the dormant cancer awakens. In some it remains asleep. I told her about reading Christiane Northrup's warning in *Women's Bodies, Women's Wisdom.* She cautions that conventional hormone replacement therapy might awaken inactive breast cancer. I told her about the research on soy and flaxseed possibly reducing breast cancer risk. Then, I couldn't help myself. I proselytized, "You really should eat some soy or flaxseed every day." Melly laughed at me. She always laughs when I get protective. She assured me, "I will. I promise. Remember, I'm the one who loves tofu. You're the one who hates it."

〰 REAPING THE BENEFITS OF PLANT ESTROGENS

I had decided to forgo hormone replacement therapy as long as my bones remained strong. Now I needed to figure out a simple system for tracking my daily plant estrogen intake. I went into chart-making mode. I summed up the soy research.

REAPING THE POTENTIAL BENEFITS OF SOY

Decrease breast cancer risk	1–2 portions
Reduce menopausal symptoms	1–2 portions
Lower cholesterol	2–5 portions
Approximate a bone-protective dose of pharmaceutical estrogen	3–8 portions

ONE PORTION OF SOY EQUALS

• 1 cup soy milk	• ⅓ cup soy flour	• ⅓ cup soybeans
• ¼ cup TVP	• 1 soyburger	• ⅓ cup dry-roasted soy nuts
• ¼ cake tofu	• 2 soy hot dogs	

I reviewed the flaxseed research. Judging from the studies, a tablespoon of flaxseed is approximately equal to a portion of soy.

REAPING THE POTENTIAL BENEFITS OF FLAXSEED	
Decrease breast cancer risk	1 tablespoon
Reduce menopausal symptoms	2–3 tablespoons
Lower cholesterol	2–5 tablespoons
Approximate a bone-protective dose of pharmaceutical estrogen	3–8 tablespoons

Seeing my personal goal in black and white—three to eight servings of soy and/or flaxseed daily—was sobering. I knew my initial enthusiasm would motivate me only for a while. I'm no different from anyone else. For a few days, a few weeks, even a few months, I could eat in a new, weird, healthy way. But if I were to continue for a long time—to make a permanent change—it would have to be easy, quick, and great-tasting. Otherwise, between Sara and Michael, my job and my friends, the shopping and the house, I wouldn't have time. I wasn't about to become a slave to the stove. Cooking with plant estrogens might have become my mission, but that mission would run out of steam if it wasn't fueled by fast, fun food.

COOKING FOR A CHANGE

Driven by a desire for easy estrogenic recipes, I rediscovered my childhood enthusiasm for culinary creation. When I was little girl, I loved to cook. Every time my parents left me alone for an hour or so, they admonished me, "Don't cook!" As soon as they were out of sight, I cooked. I couldn't resist concocting my very own original treats. Brown sugar–and–walnut candy was the best. My appetite for playing in the kitchen didn't end when I left home. At college, I stopped eating meat. My best friend, Annie, was my cooking buddy. We invented vegetarian cuisine. When I became a mother, I found a way to stay home with my children. I cooked. I wrote four cookbooks. Then, cooking became work. I burned out. I became a psychologist, and my devotion to innovative recipe making receded into the distant past. Manju, my older daughter, did her best to keep the home-cooked memories alive. She'd tell her younger sister, "Sara, you don't remember, but Mom used to cook. She even made whole-wheat cream puffs." I never thought I'd take joy in cooking again, but menopause changed me. My desire for estrogenic edibles reignited my enthusiasm for cooking.

Still, I needed a new attitude toward tofu. I began by going tofu shopping. The whole experience was like buying a mattress. There's extra-firm, firm, soft, and silken. I bought silken. It sounded the most comfortable. Once home, I opened the package. The stuff had a weird, custardlike consistency. I tasted it. It was disgusting. It tasted just like . . . tofu. But I couldn't get over the fact that it *looked* like custard. Operating on the conviction that chocolate cures anything, I decided to make it into chocolate pudding. I dumped the silken stuff into the food processor with a bunch of cocoa powder, threw in some maple syrup, and added a lot of vanilla. I blended it. I tasted it. I loved it. Unbelievable—I really loved it.

From that moment on, I began thinking of tofu as an ingredient, not a food. It's like flour. I never say, "I hate flour." I don't explain, "I only like my flour fried with soy sauce." I wouldn't ask, "Do you really like flour?" And you wouldn't answer, "Only with enough vegetables to hide the taste." Of course not! Flour is a useful ingredient. Nobody expects flour to taste good. Tofu is a useful ingredient. Why should I expect it to taste good?

So that's my transformational tofu realization. *"It's not how tofu tastes straight out of the package that matters, it's what I can do with the stuff."*

Tofu enabled me to indulge my insatiable desire for creamy food. Years earlier, I had banished the cream cheese, heavy cream, and sour cream from my diet. Now, with tofu in my life, the creamy stuff came back, but without the cream—cheesecakes, mousse cakes, puddings, custards, and sorbets; cherry-filled blintzes, wild-mushroom omelets, salmon soufflé, spinach quiche, lox-and-onion scrambles; pâtés and dips; chowders and creamy soups; pasta with roasted-pepper cream sauce, basil cream sauce, or smoked-mackerel cream sauce. All the while, I was increasing my protein intake and lowering my calorie count. I loved it. I felt like I had beaten the system.

I found flaxseed at the health food store. Disguised as the perfect bird food, these mighty mites among plant estrogen foods are a bargain. I got queenly quantities of little dark-brown seeds for a pauper's price.

I decided to grind them up with a bit of salt in my coffee grinder. I sprinkled the newly formed flax salt on my food. It tasted just fine. I ground some more, added honey and cinnamon, and sprinkled it over cooked apple slices—violà! Apple crumble. From there the recipes came easily—graham cracker–type crusts, crunchy cereals, granola, breakfast bars. All without added oil!

I dreamed and schemed. Flaxseed and soybeans filled my fantasy life, dancing through my mind, turning into snacks and treats. I was back in the kitchen again, transformed into a mad kitchen chemist. For weeks, months, and on to a year, I traveled between the natural food store and the stove, experimenting, inventing, and eating.

≋ MY PERSONAL PLANT ESTROGEN PROGRAM

I concentrated on my own "fast fun food"—munchables and desserts. I surprised myself by coming up with recipes that packed multiple portions of plant estrogens in every serving. In the morning, if I wanted breakfast, I fed myself a bowl of crunchy cereal with soy milk. In one sitting I spooned six or seven portions of plant estrogen into my menopausal body. On other days when I was too lazy to cook, I got eight portions of soy and flaxseed by eating two snack bars and drinking two 16-ounce mugs of steaming spiced soy milk. When I was more motivated, I made up tasty treats. A cool, creamy shake or a slice of mousse cake gave me three portions of plant estrogen. I found simple ways to get all the potential benefits—to reduce my risk of breast cancer, lower my cholesterol, minimize my hot flashes, and protect my bones—by eating delicious munchables. I loved my new food!

I started playing my own little game of "hide the soy, hide the flax." I asked Michael and Sara, "How much soy do you think is in this creamy soup?" They guessed. I answered, "More than two servings in each bowl!" "How much in the pasta?" "At least one." "How much in the vegetables?" "About one." "How much in the dessert?" "More than two portions in just one piece." Finally Sara got sick of humoring her estrogen-obsessed mother. Rolling her eyes as only an adolescent can, she made a reasonable request: "Please. Stop. I like the food. It's fine. I don't mind that every meal is a new and improved disguise for soybeans and flaxseed. I'm glad you're getting your plant estrogen. I'm happy you're feeding me well. I think you're a good mother. I think you're a great cook. But please, can we make a rule? Can we just eat the food without talking about it? Can you keep your calculations to yourself?"

I obeyed. I kept my calculations to myself. But tracking how many portions of plant estrogen I ate in a day became my personal project. Snack bars, shakes, and cereals gave me more than two portions of plant estrogen in every serving. Soups, main dishes, and desserts provided more than one portion. I made a list of options and combinations I could eat to tap into the potential benefits.

To decrease breast cancer risk, eat any one of the following in one day:
- One serving of almost any breakfast, soup, lunch, dinner, or dessert recipe
- Two servings of nearly every instant-estrogen recipe—mayonnaise, sprinkles, syrups, and sauces

To reduce menopausal symptoms, including hot flashes and vaginal dryness, eat any one of the following in one day:
- One breakfast bar
- One shake plus one sandwich with soy mayonnaise
- One soup plus one salad
- One main dish plus one dessert

To protect cardiovascular health, eat any one of the following in one day:
- One breakfast bar
- One soup and salad
- One main dish and one dessert
- Two cups hot spiced soy milk and two tablespoons flax sprinkle

To lower cholesterol, eat any one of the following in one day:
- One crunchy cereal with milk

- One eggless omelet with hot spiced soy milk
- One serving crêpes with creme filling
- One creamy soup, one salad, and one soy-nut snack
- One main dish, one side dish, and one custard

To approximate a standard dose of pharmaceutical estrogen, eat any one of the following in one day:
- One Maple-Nut or Malted Cereal with soy milk
- Two flax bars, two cups of hot spiced soy milk, and one main dish
- One crunchy cereal, one snack bar, and one vegetable dish
- One eggless omelet, one soup, one flax bar, and one dessert
- One serving pancakes with syrup, one thick creamy shake, and one flax bar
- One soup, one main dish, one vegetable side dish, one salad, one dessert, and one cup spiced soy milk

Some of the recipes, particularly those for breakfast foods, turned out to contain enormous quantities of plant estrogen. I had difficulty containing my enthusiasm. I kept a list of the all-time winners.

RECIPES WITH THE MOST PLANT ESTROGEN PER SERVING

Maple-Nut Crunch	8 portions plant estrogen per serving
Malted Cinnamon Crunch	8 portions plant estrogen per serving
Cinnamon-Malt Granola	4 portions plant estrogen per serving
Date-Nut Granola	4 portions plant estrogen per serving
New England Maple-Cranberry Granola	4 portions plant estrogen per serving
Lemon-Blueberry Pancakes	4 portions plant estrogen per serving
Swedish Oatmeal Pancakes	4 portions plant estrogen per serving
Rice-Wheat Pancakes	4 portions plant estrogen per serving
Apple-Orange Pancakes	4 portions plant estrogen per serving
Trail Mix	3⅔ portions plant estrogen per serving
Puffed Corn Ball Trail Mix	3⅔ portions plant estrogen per serving
Strawberry Crêpes	3½ portions plant estrogen per serving
Apple-Orange Blintzes	3½ portions plant estrogen per serving
Peanut Butter–Nut Bars	3 portions plant estrogen per serving
Buckwheat Pancakes	3 portions plant estrogen per serving

I kept the most powerfully packed plant estrogen recipes to myself. They were my menopausal food—my own alternative to hormone replacement. But not all my recipes remained my personal property.

Michael demanded his share. He was sitting on the couch reading *Time* magazine, the April 1, 1996, issue with General Norman Schwarzkopf on the cover. He looked up and announced, "I want to eat more of your food." I was surprised. I asked, "Why?" He explained, "I keep reading that soy prevents prostate cancer. It says here one in five American men will get prostate cancer. Michael Milken eats a ton of soy because he believes it's prostate-cancer protective. I know I've been making jokes about my voice going up an octave from eating your estrogen-filled food, but prostate cancer makes me nervous." I needed clarification. "So, you want to eat more soy? Do you want to eat more flaxseed too?" He answered, "Yes. I want both." He showed me a book he'd been reading—*Optimum Sports Nutrition* by Michael Colgan. "Everything I read tells me flax is really good for men. It's supposed to lower cholesterol." I was pleased. It meant I could cook estrogen-rich meals for the whole family. Still, I wanted to keep some food for myself. I told him, "You can't eat all my maple-nut crunch." He assured me, "I don't want your maple-nut crunch. I need only one or two portions a day. More might be too much."

Even Sara, my teenage daughter, wanted her share. She'd come home from school, open the fridge, and yell in a slightly accusatory tone, "Mom, did you eat all the tofu stuff? You didn't leave any of the chocolate mousse cake for me? Will you make me some cherry custard?" Actually, I was glad to make her cherry custard. My daughters have Michael's genes. His parents suffer from dangerously high blood pressure and seriously high cholesterol. If a little soy could lessen their future risk, I'd make cherry custard every day.

SEEDS OF CHANGE

Two weeks into my new plant estrogen–rich diet, I started noticing subtle changes. I began to feel more comfortable. My temperature still rose astronomically, but the sensation was different. I was still hot, but the heat wasn't preceded by this creepy-crawly feeling all over my skin. I felt more comfortable, less physically and emotionally agitated. After three weeks, my night sweats turned into hot flashes. I was waking, but I wasn't drenched in sweat.

Six weeks went by. Sometimes I had one hot flash a day; sometimes none. I woke up just once a night, overheating for only a few minutes. I become more rested, craved less caffeine, and took less aspirin.

Eight weeks went by. I woke up one morning and it was light outside. I felt disoriented. I asked Michael, "What happened?" He said, "What do you mean 'What happened?'?" I told him, "I don't remember the night." He explained, "Most people don't remember the night. Most people sleep through the night." "That's what happened," I announced. Now *he* was confused. "What? What are you talking about?" I said, "That's what happened. I slept through the night." He understood. He asked me, "How long has it been since you slept through the night?" I thought about it before I answered: "Nearly a year." He asked for details: "No sweats?" I answered, "No sweats. I'm completely rested. I feel so incredibly good." He advised caution. "It's just one night. Don't get your expectations up." I reminded myself, "I'm taking care of myself for the long-term benefits. Given my family history, I can't expect estrogenic eating to rid me of menopausal heat waves."

Michael was right. The next two nights, I woke up once each night.

Then I slept through the night again. This time, I woke up quietly. Hearing the birds sing, feeling our bed bathed in morning light, I appreciated the moment. Another night came and passed with eight hours of uninterrupted slumber. Two nights in a row! What pleasure! Then, three nights. Now, four nights! Five. Six. An entire week of sleep-filled nights. I asked myself, "When was the last time you had a hot flash?" I couldn't remember. Nor could I recall my last headache.

Three months went by without a hot flash or a night sweat. Then I made a mistake. I got cocky. I thought, "I must be different from my mom and my grandmother. I must be finished with menopause." I got a little lax about my diet. Within a week, I woke up too hot to sleep. I passed it off as a one-night thing. The next night I woke up sweating. I reinstituted my dietary routine. Within a week, my night sweats disappeared again. I lectured myself, "You can't afford to take a vacation from taking care of your body."

As a year went by, my oversensitive thermostat taught me two lessons:

- If you drink too much caffeine, your menopausal body will heat up.
- If you don't eat your flaxseed and soy, your temperature will rise.

On my fiftieth birthday, I gave a party—a small party. I invited only old friends—friends I'd known for half my life and expected to know for the rest of our lives. Martin came. You remember. He's the acupuncturist and Chinese herbalist I trust completely. I asked for a checkup. He felt my pulses for several minutes, then said, "Last year you had the pulses of a menopausal woman. This year you have the pulses of a premenopausal woman." I asked, "Is that good?" He nodded. "That's very good." I asked, "What should I do now?" He answered, "Just keep doing what you're doing. It's working."

At my next checkup, my doctor agreed: "Your bones are holding up well. You're not showing the usual signs of postmenopausal dryness. Your breasts are normal. Your blood pressure's still low. And your cholesterol count couldn't be better."

It's been more than four years since I began eating estrogenically. I'm no longer so alone. Even *Obstetrics & Gynecology*, the journal of the American College of Obstetricians and Gynecologists, is considering the possibility that foods rich in plant estrogens may benefit those of us in the throes of hormonal upheaval. In the May 1996 issue, Knight and Eden reviewed 861 medical articles and concluded that estrogen-rich foods offer a "safe, cheap, generally side-effect-free alternative to current pharmaceutical measures."

That's my story. No doubt your story is different. You have different risk factors. Different sensibilities. Different concerns. You'll make your own estrogen decision. No one, not even your doctor, certainly not me, can make that decision for you. You'll think and worry and investigate. You'll seek safe passage in your own way. If you decide to include plant estrogens in your plans, I hope this book will be helpful. I hope you enjoy new adventures in shopping, cooking, and eating.

Two

The Plant Estrogen Pantry

When you start packing your pantry with plant estrogen–rich foods, the look of your grocery cart will change. Mine is regularly packed with twelve cakes of tofu, six half gallons of soy milk, two packages of soy-dogs, one pack of soyburgers, a tube of ground soy "meat," and five 1-pound bags of flaxseed. Let me warn you, this unusual grocery order could cause you some embarrassment at the checkout counter. Like the day I decided to be honest about my menopausal condition with the grocery clerk.

I stacked my four packages of silken tofu, two of soft tofu, three of firm tofu, and three of extra-firm tofu on the checkout counter. As they rolled by, the cashier—a sensitive, wire-rimmed-glasses kind of guy of about forty—commented, "You eat a lot of tofu." Next I loaded the other soy products. Again he noted, "You eat a lot of soy." Then came the five bags of flaxseed. Smiling, he asked, "How do you use all this soy and flaxseed?" Eager to share my newfound adventure, I answered, "I eat them all the time, in practically everything. They're loaded with plant estrogen." At the word estrogen, he averted his eyes. Suddenly the electric scanner demanded his total attention. I'm certain I saw him gulp. I think he blushed. I chided myself, "Oh, no. You embarrassed him. He knows you need estrogen. He knows you're going through menopause. For him it's like you're standing in the middle of this respectable grocery store yelling very loudly, 'Hey, look at me. I'm drying up fast. I need lubrication.' " He continued attending exclusively to each bag of flaxseed, passing it carefully over the scanner, making it emanate the perfect beep. I watched. He didn't look at me again. I wanted to answer his question in detail—to tell him how I used all this soy and flaxseed—but he really didn't want to know. Now, I'll tell you instead.

≋ TOFU

You can find tofu in almost any supermarket these days. Tofu is a white block of soy "cheese"—actually made from soy milk. It's sold immersed in water in 16- to 19-ounce packages. In Chinese and Thai cuisine, tofu is cut into pieces and added to vegetable dishes. In Japan, tofu takes many forms, from the common blocks of tofu to delicate, thin tofu skin. The Japanese consider cooking with tofu an art form.

Nutritionally, tofu, even without its plant estrogen content, is an extraordinary food. In a ½-cup serving you get about 10 grams of protein and only 90 calories. If it's made with calcium sulfate, it will give you 553 mg of calcium in a serving. That's a third to a half of the recommended calcium intake for a menopausal women. Along with the protein and calcium, tofu also gives you iron, zinc, and B vitamins.

As you probably know by now, I hate the taste of tofu. Other cookbooks will tell you, "Tofu is a chameleon. It reflects the flavor of other foods and spices." Don't believe them. Tofu doesn't reflect. It absorbs. It sucks up all the flavoring you throw at it. It refuses to taste like anything except tofu until it eats up massive amounts of herbs, spices, or extracts. Cinnamon, cardamom, nutmeg, dill, and basil are packed with calcium. So don't be shy. Throw them into tofu dishes by the tablespoonful. Or add almond, vanilla, orange, or lemon extract a spoonful at a time. Tofu will stubbornly refuse to yield to their influence. Then, at some magical point, a transformation occurs. Tofu becomes something else. It becomes edible—even enjoyable. It becomes good food.

Despite my distaste for the soy flavor of tofu, I've become a tofu-dependent cook. Tofu has become an indispensable ingredient in my kitchen. I use it in place of flour for making sauces and gravies; in place of sour cream and cream cheese for making dips, creamy soups, pasta sauces, puddings, custards, cheesecakes, and mousses; in place of eggs to make omelets, scrambles, soufflés, and blintzes. Once you start experimenting with its potential, you'll be amazed by its versatility.

To get the very most out of tofu, you'll need an electric food processor and an electric blender. There's no need to spend a lot of money on these appliances. I bought my first food processor on sale for less than twenty dollars. It lasted fifteen years! When I bought a replacement, I paid less than thirty dollars. Blenders can cost even less.

Tofu spoils quickly if it is not stored in water. Place any unused portion in a container filled with fresh water before refrigerating. When properly stored, the unused tofu will remain fresh for a week or longer.

To get the most out of tofu, it helps to understand its different densities. There are four basic types of tofu: silken, soft, firm, and extra-firm.

Silken Tofu

Silken tofu is the most fun. It's also the lowest in fat. Whipped up in a food processor with ample flavorings or fruit, it makes the creamiest puddings, custards, cheesecakes, sauces, dressings, and soups. Not every grocery store stocks silken tofu, but it can be ordered from the same companies that make other densities of tofu.

Soft Tofu

Soft tofu is especially useful in dips and pâtés. It also has a place in cream soups, salad dressings, gravies, and sauces.

Soft tofu can be used in place of silken, but it doesn't work as well. To use soft as a silken alternative, you need to process it in an electric food processor with 2 or 3 tablespoons of liquid for 3 to 5 minutes. Patience and tolerance for noise are required. But if soft tofu is processed long enough, it will lose its graininess, take on a glossy sheen, and become custardlike.

Firm Tofu

Firm tofu absorbs flavors. It can be marinated in ginger or in sweet-and-sour or soy-based sauces. To really taste fully marinated, firm tofu needs to be soaked in sauce overnight or baked in marinade at 300°F for more than an hour.

I like firm tofu fried—deep-fried. It takes on a chewy texture. It develops this slightly crisp outer layer. It's great. The only problem is, deep-fried tofu is deep-fried. You can't take any food, no matter how healthy, boil it in fat, and expect it to be good for you. As a compromise, you can oven-roast it using canola-oil spray. Cut the firm tofu into triangles. Spray both sides of each triangle with just a bit of oil. Put them on a cookie sheet. Bake them for 10 minutes on each side in a 500°F oven. You get the crispy, chewy texture with much less fat.

Given the food-processor treatment—puréed and pulverized—firm tofu transforms itself into eggless omelets and soufflés. A dab of turmeric for color, some garlic, ginger, and mustard for taste, and voilà—*eggs!* Well, maybe not quite eggs, but a mystery food that will keep them guessing.

Extra-Firm Tofu

Extra-firm tofu is dense. It refuses to absorb flavors. Don't believe anyone who says, "Let extra-firm tofu marinate. It will absorb flavors." When will this happen? Not on my watch. It absorbs flavors in its own good time—like in three weeks.

Forget the marinade. Mash in the flavor. When you mash in minced garlic, onion, capers, sun-dried tomatoes, chives, basil, or parsley along with a little salt, soy sauce, or mustard, extra-firm tofu becomes a tasty crumbled mass. Crumbled flavored extra-firm tofu works well tossed with greens or pasta.

When extra-firm tofu is properly flavored, it makes excellent baked cheesecakes, quiches, and loaves. The transformation can be successfully accomplished without eggs or cream cheese. But it does require a full 5 minutes in the electric food processor to eliminate all stubborn grains from the tofu.

Other Tofu Products

Every time I turn my back, another tofu product pops up on the grocery shelf. They range from great to terrible. You'll need to experiment as new, improved products come along. Baked, smoked, barbecued, Cajun, Mexican, Thai, and fried—I've tried them all. Every once in a while I like one. Usually, I don't.

Tofu Mayonnaise, Dips, Cream Cheese, Ice Cream, and Ravioli

Other new foods often excite me. Ready-made tofu mayonnaise passes easily for the usual heart-stopping combo of eggs and oil. Dips with enough flavor to wipe out the taste of tofu can be spectacular. Tofutti makes a fabulous no-fat, no-cholesterol, dairy-free apple-vanilla ice cream and ice cream sandwiches. I even found some fantastic Soy Boy ravioli with sun-dried tomato–and–pesto filling.

〰 WHOLE SOYBEANS

Dried soybeans are brownish-yellow and the size of white or black-eyed beans. Boiled, ½ cup has about 15 grams of protein and 150 calories. Boiled soybeans are also a good source of vitamin A, most B vitamins, and calcium. Sometimes you can find whole dried soybeans in the bulk-food bins in natural foods stores, but they are not readily available.

There's probably a reason whole dried soybeans are hard to find. While they are indisputably nutritious, they take forever to cook. After an hour of boiling, they're still hard enough to break a tooth with every bite. Soybeans take a full eight hours of boiling before they're edible. And even when they're completely cooked, they're still hard to digest, and they have no taste. I don't use whole dried soybeans in any of my recipes.

≋ SOY NUTS

Soy nuts are soybeans that are dry-roasted until crisp; they taste like reduced-oil peanuts. A half cup has 30 grams of protein but also about 400 calories. Like dried soybeans, they provide good nutrition—vitamin A, B vitamins, and calcium. These nutty little treats are also packed with calcium—232 mg in ½ cup.

Soy nuts taste fine, but they're too dry. Tossed with a little oil and curry powder, they're perfect. Ground with salt, they make a Thai-style condiment. Mixed with hot barley malt, they turn into nut brittle. But use them in baked goods or cook them in vegetable dishes and they get soggy. I toss them on top of Chinese dishes at the last minute so they don't have a chance to soak up liquid.

≋ SOY MILK

Soy milk is a whole soybean product. It gives you all the nutrition of soybeans—protein, iron, B vitamins, and omega-3 essential fatty acids. Soy milk, like cow's milk, can be bought in nonfat, low-fat, and full-fat forms. When a soy milk container says "1 percent" on the carton, that doesn't mean 1 percent of its calories come from fat. It means it's 1 percent fat by weight! Since it contains a large amount of water, it's heavy. In reality, a carton of soy milk that brags about being 1 percent fat gets about 25 percent of its calories from fat. The same principle applies to cow's milk.

Personally, I began hating soy milk the day I was born. My mother tells the story about the very first time she fed me. She stuck a bottle of soy formula in my waiting mouth. I wrinkled my face in disgust, spit out the soy milk, and cried. Months of formula feeding led to little in-gestion and minimal weight gain. Finally, the family doctor said, "Give her real milk!" I sucked up the whole bottle with delight.

My negative attitude persisted until I discovered Silk, a soy milk made and distributed by White Wave, Inc., of Boulder, Colorado. I buy gallons of Silk every week. I actually drink it straight from the bot-tle and pour it directly over cereal! You can find it in the dairy case in a well-stocked natural foods store. White Wave products have a large dis-tribution network. Your natural foods store can easily order it for you.

In my opinion every soy milk—with the exception of Silk—tastes like watered-down soybeans. My husband disagrees. He voluntarily pours soy milk over his cereal. He says I have a bad attitude. He in-forms me, "Stores don't put soy milk on the shelves for decoration. People do buy it, drink it, and like it." If you're like me and find soy milk hard to swallow, try flavoring it with ground cardamom, cinna-mon, nutmeg, or almond extract. They improve its flavor dramatically. Soy milk is available plain, unsweetened, or flavored.

Soy milk can be used in cooking and baking in place of cow's milk. Also, soy milk acts like cow's milk in one other respect: It curdles when heated with acidic foods like lemon or tomato.

≋ SOY FLOUR

Soy flour is simply ground-up dried soybeans. It comes in two forms—raw and lightly toasted. The raw flour tastes raw—like bitter green soy-beans. The toasted is easier to digest and tastes nutty. Most of the soy flour found in stores is defatted. It's a by-product from making soy oil. A half cup contains about 23 grams of protein and 165 calories. Only 3 percent of the calories in defatted soy flour comes from fat.

Soy flour works in nearly anything baked. It can take the place of about 20 percent of the flour in most recipes. But soy flour is a glutton for water. Increasing liquid by just a little helps preserve moistness. And soy flour browns quickly. Lowering the baking temperature by about 25 degrees prevents burning.

TVP—texturized vegetable protein

The mainstream and natural foods markets are being flooded by meat-like products. TVP—texturized vegetable protein—has been around the longest. Uncooked TVP comes in the form of light-brown, hard, irregularly shaped pellets made by extracting the protein from soybeans. It can be found in natural foods stores in packages or in bulk. But for those of us looking for plant estrogens, TVP is an undependable source. According to Stephen Barnes, Ph.D., a well-respected soy researcher, the plant estrogen in TVP can be destroyed in processing. If the protein is extracted using a water process, the plant estrogen remains intact. If the protein is extracted using an alcohol process, the plant estrogen tends to be destroyed. In either case, the protein in TVP is impressive—16.3 grams in just 1 ounce with only 1 percent fat.

Thrown into chili, it's a good low-fat, high-fiber substitute for hamburger. As for making hamburger-type patties, I can never make it work. The texture's never right. They come out too soggy or spongy or crunchy.

Soy Burgers, Soy Ground "Meats," and Soy Hot Dogs

Some factories, big and small, produce excellent soy "meats." Lightlife Foods, for example, makes great hamburgerlike and sausagelike foods. Their fat-free hot dogs—Smart Dogs—really do taste like all-beef franks. Lightlife assures me their protein isolate is water-extracted. The result is high-protein, fat-free, plant estrogen–rich products.

Soy meats cook exactly like their flesh-food counterparts. They can be fried, broiled, barbecued, or baked.

≋ TEMPEH

Tempeh is fermented whole soybeans. As a plant estrogen source, it's a bit controversial. On the basis of population studies, some researchers seem to think that fermented soybeans are not as likely to reduce breast cancer risk. However, Andrea Hutchins, Ph.D., reports in the *Journal of the American Dietetic Association* that the plant estrogen in fermented products may actually be more available to the body than that in non-fermented products. Tempeh has a chewy texture that some people relish. I find it difficult to eat. To me it looks too unappetizing.

Tempeh can be used and cooked in the same way as meat-mimicking products. I have not been able to develop a taste for it, so none of my recipes call for tempeh.

≋ MISO

Miso is soybean paste. It can be found in the refrigerated section of most natural foods stores. The soybeans are fermented and aged until they form a dense brown paste. Miso comes in different shades of brown. Dark-brown miso is concentrated pure soybeans—high in plant estrogens. The lighter colors combine grains with soy. The combination cuts the plant estrogen content and sweetens the taste.

Dark-brown miso makes a great bouillon—just stir it into hot water to taste. It also works well as a stock base for any soup calling for beef stock. Lighter-colored misos are used in traditional miso soup. Just dissolve in hot water and add a little cut-up tofu. The lighter, sweeter miso gives borscht, salad dressings, and sauces a sweet and salty taste. In many recipes miso can be used instead of salt.

≋ SOY PROTEIN POWDERS AND SOY SUPPLEMENTS

It's a shame. It's a sham.

In the vitamin section of natural foods stores, you will find protein powders and soy pills. The labels may claim to be "rich in phytonutrients" and "filled with isoflavones"—more technical terms for plant estrogens. Be careful. Most protein powders are stripped of plant estrogens. Even those that claim to be different may be misleading. For example: One product declares itself to be a women's health product filled with phytoestrogens. It reads, "18 milligrams isoflavone per serving." According to Mark Messina, Ph.D., a cup of soy milk has more than 40 mg of phytoestrogens. If you're looking for plant estrogens, forget the protein powder. Just use whole soy products as part of a balanced diet.

Soy pills can be equally deceptive. When you read the fine print, you'll often find that one tablet contains 12 mg. That means you'd need to take three tablets to equal a quarter cake of tofu. What a deal! You get none of the protein, none of the calcium, none of the B vitamins, and one third the plant estrogens for two or three times the price!

≋ FLAXSEED

What are flaxseeds? To find out, I consulted encyclopedias and nutrition almanacs. Flaxseeds are dark-brown seeds, the size of sesame seeds. They have a pleasant nutty taste. While not a common food in our culture, flax has a long history. People throughout the world have grown flaxseed—also called linseed—from time immemorial. The ancients wove the plant fibers into cloth, paper, and rope. The Egyptians used the cloth for wrapping mummies. Even today, furniture enthusiasts use flaxseed oil to maintain their most valued possessions. Flaxseed was also one of the first food crops ever grown. People have been consuming flax for 5,000 years. Today, people in Scandinavia, Africa, and Asia eat flaxseed regularly. This food isn't an experimental substance used only in laboratories and by food faddists.

Flaxseed contains about 18 percent protein. Three tablespoons of seed have 75.9 mg of calcium and about 300 mg of potassium. The seed also contains iron and B vitamins. A 3-tablespoon serving contains 15 percent of the recommended daily minimum of iron, 2 percent of niacin, 4 percent of thiamine, and 4 percent of riboflavin. In addition, flaxseed contains boron, one of those newly touted, hard-to-get micronutrients. According to Forrest Neilson, Ph.D., of the United

States Department of Agriculture, preliminary investigations suggest that boron may be essential for bone strength and may even have some estrogenic effects.

Let me take a moment to remind you about the estrogenic potency of flaxseed. In laboratory experiments, the type of plant estrogen in flax—called *lignans*—has a more noticeable estrogenic effect than soy-plant estrogens—called *isoflavones*. Laboratory analysis of flaxseed done at the University of Toronto showed that flaxseed has between 75 and 800 times more lignans than any other food.

Even before researchers uncovered the estrogenic qualities of flax-seed, alternative-medicine enthusiasts used it for two purposes—heart health and digestive regularity. In *Spontaneous Healing*, Andrew Weil, M.D., recommends consuming 2 tablespoons of ground flaxseed daily to benefit the cardiovascular system. Naturopathic practitioners often recommend flaxseed to alleviate the discomforts of constipation.

Flaxseed is high in soluble fiber—the same kind of fiber found in oatmeal. If you soak flaxseed in water overnight, you'll find it turns into a gelatinous mass. The fiber actually begins to dissolve. The ability of flaxseed to thicken water makes it a particularly gentle fiber and an amazing baking ingredient.

Baking and Cooking with Flaxseed

Flaxseed can add moisture and lightness to baked goods. Vegans—they eat no meat, eggs, or dairy products—use flaxseed in much of their baking. In *Recipes from an Ecological Kitchen*, Lorna J. Sass recommends 1 tablespoon of flaxseed blended in an electric blender with 2 tablespoons of water in place of one egg. In Finland, flaxseed bread is a staple of the daily diet. A few tablespoons are kneaded into nearly every loaf.

This conversion is dependable, but it doesn't give you a lot of plant estrogens in every serving. To lace baked goods with more lignans is a bit tricky. If you add too much flaxseed to cookies, brownies, cakes, breads, or pancakes, they will becomes overmoist—gooey inside. But if you get the proportions just right, the results are quite incredible. You can have moist, light baked goods with no added oil or eggs. I follow two guidelines:

- Use at least two to three times as much flour as flaxseed.
- Bake at a low temperature for at least twice as long as a conventional recipe calls for.

Flaxseed-rich baked goods stay moist longer than their conventional counterparts, but they should be refrigerated between servings. Otherwise, their internal moisture attracts mold—particularly in hot, humid weather. It's hard to produce leavened baked goods—those made with baking soda, baking powder, or yeast—with flaxseed, but you can't go wrong when you make flaxseed fruit crisps, graham cracker–type crusts, crunchy cereals, granolas, and snack bars. When made with flaxseed, all these foods—normally high in fat—require no added oil. Nearly all can be made using all-fruit preserves or fruit-juice concentrates—no sugar, no empty calories. Most give you multiple portions of plant estrogen in deliciously decadent forms.

To make flax cereals, crusts, and snack bars, you will need a small electric coffee grinder. You can easily grind ⅓ to ½ cup of seeds at a time. Grinding them fresh for each recipe takes just seconds. Once ground, flaxseed can lose its nutrients quickly. It's therefore best to keep all your flaxseed concoctions refrigerated.

Flaxseed can be found in vacuum-packed 1-pound packages in most natural foods stores. If your store does not carry flaxseed, the store manager can order it from a major distributor of grains and flours—Arrowhead Mills in Hereford, Texas. Since flaxseed is an oil seed, it can go rancid. It's best to store open packages in the refrigerator.

≋ FLAX POWDER

Not a Cooking Ingredient!

Flaxseed powder is an expensive by-product of flax-oil production. Because most of the oil is removed, it's about 13 percent fat. This gray-brown grainy flour is used primarily as a laxative. But if you consume flaxseed powder without drinking large amounts of water, it causes stomach distress.

Flaxseed powder might seem to be a time-saving alternative to grinding flaxseed one batch at a time. It's not! The powder soaks up enormous amounts of liquid, coagulating quickly and forming a rubbery ball. It transforms nearly any recipe into an indigestible mass.

≋ FLAX OIL

Flax oil is scary. If you forget to keep it cold, it will literally turn into furniture polish. When it's fresh, flax oil tastes slightly nutty. When it begins to age, it tastes bitter, like orange peel. When it's old, it tastes like fish oil. At that point, it can give you indigestion, even cause vomiting. Fresh flax oil can be found in natural foods stores. Be certain to buy only refrigerated oil in opaque bottles. The best flax oil will always have an expiration date on the bottle.

Despite its fragility, flax oil is highly touted by many health practitioners. They recommend a tablespoon or more a day as a supplemental source of omega-3 essential fatty acids, which are widely reported to have cardiovascular benefits.

Contrary to some reports, flax oil is *not* a good source of the plant estrogens called *lignans*. When flax oil is pressed out of flaxseed, the plant estrogens do not remain in the oil. They stay with the residue—the flax powder. At least one company advertises its product as "high-lignan flax oil." In reality, the lignan content of this oil is meager compared to flaxseed. After removing the oil, 15 to 18 percent of the lignan-containing residue is reintroduced into the oil. To put it another way, you would need to take 5 or 6 tablespoons of "high-lignan" flax oil to get the same amount of plant estrogens in 1 tablespoon of flaxseed.

Nevertheless, used sparingly, high-lignan flax oil can be a useful addition to some recipes. Salad dressings and pasta sauces sometimes cry out for just a touch more oil. In these cases, I do use a little flax oil because of its potential health benefits.

Remember not to heat flax oil. You should avoid cooking or baking with it. High temperatures will hasten its demise, making it rancid. In rare cases, it could even make you feel sick.

≋ THE COMPLETE PANTRY

While flaxseed and soy products form the basis of a diet rich in plant estrogens, a complete menopausal diet needs to include a variety of natural foods. Fruits, vegetables, and whole grains provide indispensable nutrition. Spices, herbs, and seeds often contain surprisingly high quantities of calcium. Dried fruit, fruit juice concentrates, and all-fruit jams provide goodly amounts of the mineral boron, now thought to contribute to bone maintenance and menopausal health. Some people may be allergic to soy or flaxseed. If your body rebels against any food, respect that reaction: Stay away from it. And if you're taking medication regularly—any medication including hormone replacement therapy—be sure to speak with your doctor about making dietary changes. Please don't neglect any aspect of your health or any part of a balanced diet as you consider taking your fill of foods rich in plant estrogens.

Three

Munchables

These are fun foods—snack bars, hot steamy drinks, cold creamy shakes, and handfuls of nutty treats—all packed with multiple portions of plant estrogen. When you're trying to infuse every bite you eat with estrogenic goodness, munchables like these become basic foodstuffs. Need breakfast on the run? Grab a snack bar and you've eaten two or three portions of plant estrogen. Want to sip a big mug of hot something while you work? A steaming, flavored, creamy drink will give you another two estrogen portions. How about a creamy shake and some nutty snacks for couch-potato time? You'll get four or five portions of plant estrogen with your decadent indulgence. Just munch away. Decrease your risk of breast cancer, diminish your menopausal symptoms, lower your cholesterol, and maybe even protect your bones without ever making an estrogenic meal!

That's another great thing about munchables—they're personal-portion food. You don't have to make them for anyone else. You don't have to endure any mealtime commentary from husbands, partners, or children. You don't have to place your estrogenic concoctions on the table. You don't have to watch the apprehension on their faces. You don't have to listen to the males in your life ask, "Will my voice go up an octave?" You won't hear your children ask, "Is this more of your weird food, Mom?" You can just munch away in your own good time. You can wait for them to ask, "Did you make any snack bars?" "Why didn't you make me a shake?" "Where's my hot spiced milk?" If you don't want to share, you have the perfect excuse: "I need this snack. It's my estrogen!"

≋ SNACK BARS

I first called these fun bars "breakfast bars" because I ate them for breakfast. On weekdays, I'm just not much of a breakfast eater. About ten o'clock, I grab two bars and get an automatic four portions of plant estrogen. These breakfast substitutes give me instant energy. More than any other one food, these bars keep me cool. I eat them and no hot flashes, no night sweats. They're like delayed air-conditioning. A week of munching them for breakfast and I'm complaining about the cold— begging to keep the heat on through the chilly winter nights. If I forget to eat them for a week, I'm transported back to Sweatsville, piling all the comforters onto my husband.

Why are these bars so magical for me? All are densely packed with fresh-ground flaxseed—probably the most potent source of plant estrogen and omega-3 essential fatty acids in existence. The fruit-flax bars have an added plus. Both flaxseed and dried fruit turn out to be great sources of the mineral boron. Some reports will have you believe that boron alone will up your estrogen levels and decrease your calcium excretion. I called an expert—Dr. Forrest Neilson of the United States Department of Agriculture. He's the man the promoters of boron most often quote. I asked him, "Will boron really decrease calcium excretion by 40 percent?" He replied, "We got that result only in our first study. I think other factors helped cause the effect. We've never gotten that kind of dramatic result again." I asked, "Will it up the estrogen levels of postmenopausal women?" He explained, "The women in our study who were taking estrogen pills showed signs of utilizing the hormone more efficiently. The women who were not taking estrogen showed no predictable results." I told him my story. As soon as I said, "I'm eating lots of soy and flax for the plant estrogens," he interrupted me. "Soy is one of the best sources of boron. And flaxseed is very rich in boron also." I volunteered, "My hot flashes have pretty much disappeared. Do you think the plant estrogens and boron work together to up my estrogen level?" He commented without making a commitment, "It makes sense." We chatted about how eating food was better than taking supplements, since whole foods have so many hidden nutrients that complement one another. He promised to send me his articles. I thanked him and left our conversation feeling that boron couldn't be bad. It's worth recommending.

At first glance, snack bars may seem complicated to prepare. After making them a time or two, however, they turn into a 15-minute project. If you find them as cooling and energizing as I do, you'll whip up a batch every few days.

DATE-NUT BREAKFAST BARS

Work and Cooking Time: *under 20 minutes*
Equipment: *electric coffee grinder and electric food processor*
Yield: *Makes 8 bars*

Chewy, energy-imparting snacks—these are a date lover's dream.

¾ cup frozen apple juice concentrate
1½ cups pitted dates

1 cup flaxseed
½ cup chopped walnuts

1. Place the apple juice concentrate and dates in a saucepan. Cover and cook over medium-high heat for 5 minutes, until softened.

2. While the dates cook, grind the flaxseed in an electric coffee grinder ⅓ cup at a time. Pour the ground seeds into a food processor with the S blade inserted. Add the dates. Process until the mixture is doughlike. If the mixture rises above the processor

blades, shut off the machine and push the mixture down with a spatula. Then, turn the machine back on.

3. Pour into a bowl and mix in the walnuts.

4. Turn the dough into a 9×9-inch cake pan and press flat with damp hands to cover the entire bottom of the pan evenly. Cut into eight bars. (Make three evenly spaced cuts in one direction and one in the other.)

5. Remove from the pan. Place in a storage container or in plastic sandwich bags. Refrigerate.

PLANT ESTROGEN ESTIMATE: **2** PORTIONS PER BAR

MOLASSES-APPLE-NUT SNACK BARS

Work and Cooking Time: *under 15 minutes*
Equipment: *electric coffee grinder and electric food processor*
Yield: *Makes 8 bars*

Flavored like gingerbread, these spicy delights have a chewy texture. The blackstrap molasses and cinnamon give a calcium boost to this boron-rich, estrogen-packed snack food.

This is a good snack to eat right away. In time the soy nuts absorb moisture from the dried fruit and loose their crispiness.

¾ cup frozen apple juice concentrate

2 cups dried apples

1 cup flaxseed

1 teaspoon blackstrap molasses

2 tablespoons ground cinnamon

2 teaspoons ground ginger

1¼ cups soy nuts

1. Place the apple juice concentrate and dried apple rings in a saucepan. Cover and cook over medium-high heat for 5 minutes, until softened.

2. While the apples cook, grind the flaxseed in an electric coffee grinder ⅓ cup at a time. Pour the ground seeds into a food processor with the S blade inserted.

3. Add the molasses, cinnamon, and ginger to the food processor. By now the dried apples should be softened but should still retain their form. Add them to the food processor. Set aside ¼ cup soy nuts. Add 1 cup soy nuts.

4. Process until the mixture is doughlike and the apples are coarsely chopped. If the mixture rises above the processor blades, shut off the machine and push the mixture down with a spatula. Then, turn the machine back on.

5. Grind 2 tablespoons of the soy nuts in the coffee grinder and sprinkle half over the bottom of a 9×9-inch cake pan. Turn the dough into the pan and press flat with damp hands to cover the entire bottom of the pan evenly. Grind the remaining 2 tablespoons soy nuts and sprinkle over the flattened dough.

6. Cut into eight bars. (Make three evenly spaced cuts in one direction and one in the other.) Remove from the pan. Place in a storage container or in plastic sandwich bags. Refrigerate.

PLANT ESTROGEN ESTIMATE: 2½ PORTIONS PER BAR

CRANBERRY SNACK BARS

Work and Cooking Time: *under 20 minutes*
Equipment: *electric coffee grinder and electric food processor*
Yield: *Makes 8 bars*

Ocean Spray distributes dried cranberries. They're a fabulous food—sweet, sour, and chewy. Ocean Spray is mainstream. With prodding, any grocery store manager can stock them.

½ cup frozen cherry juice or apple juice
    concentrate

2 cups dried cranberries
1¼ cups flaxseed

1. Place the juice concentrate and dried cranberries in a saucepan. Cover and cook over medium-high heat for 5 minutes, until softened.

2. While the cranberries cook, grind the flaxseed in an electric coffee grinder ⅓ cup at a time. Pour the ground seeds into a food processor with the S blade inserted. Add the softened dried cranberries.

3. Process until the mixture is doughlike. If the mixture rises above the processor blades, shut off the machine and push the mixture down with a spatula. Then, turn the machine back on. When the dough is fully mixed, it will form a ball in the well of the food processor.

4. Press the dough evenly into a 9×9-inch nonstick or glass pan. Cut into eight bars. (Make three evenly spaced cuts in one direction, and one in the other.)

5. Remove from the pan. Place in a storage container or in plastic sandwich bags. Refrigerate.

PLANT ESTROGEN ESTIMATE: **2½ PORTIONS PER BAR**

VARIATION: *To vary the taste and texture, add ½ cup chopped walnuts.*
SUBSTITUTION: *Dried cherries can be substituted for cranberries.*

APPLE BARS

Work and Cooking Time: *under 20 minutes*
Equipment: *electric coffee grinder and electric food processor*
Yield: *Makes 8 bars*

Choose apple or orange flavor for these simplest of dried-fruit breakfast or snack bars. Either taste packs estrogenic goodness and heart-healthy omega-3s.

½ cup frozen apple juice or orange juice concentrate
2 cups dried apples

1¼ cups flaxseed
1 tablespoon vanilla extract

1. Place the juice concentrate and dried apple rings in a saucepan. Cover and cook over medium-high heat for 5 minutes, until softened.

2. While the apples cook, grind the flaxseed in an electric coffee grinder ⅓ cup at a time. Pour the ground seeds into a food processor with the S blade inserted. Add the softened dried apples and vanilla.

3. Process until the mixture is doughlike. If the mixture rises above the processor blades, shut off the machine and push the mixture down with a spatula. Then, turn the machine back on. When the dough is fully mixed, it will form a ball in the well of the food processor.

4. Press the dough evenly into a 9×9-inch cake pan. Cut into eight bars. (Make three evenly spaced cuts in one direction and one in the other.) Remove from the pan. Place in a storage container or in plastic sandwich bags. Refrigerate.

PLANT ESTROGEN ESTIMATE: 2½ PORTIONS PER BAR

ORANGE-APRICOT BARS

Work and Cooking Time: *under 20 minutes*
Equipment: *electric coffee grinder and electric food processor*
Yield: *Makes 8 bars*

Brightly colored and softly chewy, these highly estrogenic, omega-3–saturated bars are especially fruity.

2 tablespoons frozen orange juice concentrate	1½ cups flaxseed
⅓ cup frozen apple juice concentrate	1 teaspoon grated orange rind
2 cups dried apricots	

1. Place the juice concentrates and dried apricots in a saucepan. Cover and cook over medium-high heat for 5 minutes, until softened.

2. While the apricots cook, grind the flaxseed in an electric coffee grinder ⅓ cup at a time. Pour the ground seeds into a food processor with the S blade inserted. Add the softened dried apricots and the orange rind.

3. Process until the mixture is doughlike. If the mixture rises above the processor blades, shut off the machine and push the mixture down with a spatula. Then, turn the

machine back on. When the dough is fully mixed, it will form a ball in the well of the food processor.

4. Press the dough evenly into a 9×9-inch cake pan. Cut into eight bars. (Make three evenly spaced cuts in one direction and one in the other.) Remove from the pan. Place in a storage container or in plastic sandwich bags. Refrigerate.

PLANT ESTROGEN ESTIMATE: 3 PORTIONS PER BAR

PEACHY PECAN BARS

Work and Cooking Time: *under 20 minutes*
Equipment: *electric coffee grinder and electric food processor*
Yield: *Makes 8 bars*

Even in winter, these snack bars remind me of summer—they're just so peachy. Peaches are near the top of the list of boron-containing foods. When they're dried, you get the mineral in concentrated form, along with the ever-present fabulous flax duo—plant estrogens and omega-3s.

½ cup frozen grape juice concentrate
2 cups dried peaches

1¼ cups flaxseed
⅓ cup chopped pecans

1. Place the grape juice concentrate and dried peaches in a saucepan. Cover and cook over medium-high heat for 5 minutes, until softened.

2. While the peaches cook, grind the flaxseed in an electric coffee grinder ⅓ cup at a time. Pour the ground seeds into a food processor with the S blade inserted. Add the softened dried peaches.

3. Process until the mixture is doughlike. If the mixture rises above the processor blades, shut off the machine and push the mixture down with a spatula. Then, turn the machine back on. When the dough is fully mixed, it will form a ball in the well of the food processor.

4. Press half of the dough into a 9×9-inch nonstick pan. Sprinkle with the pecans. Press the remaining half of the dough over the pecans. Cut into eight bars. (Make three evenly spaced cuts in one direction and one in the other.) Remove from the pan. Place in a storage container or in plastic sandwich bags. Refrigerate.

PLANT ESTROGEN ESTIMATE: 2½ PORTIONS PER BAR

CHOCOLATE SNACK BARS

Work and Cooking Time: *under 20 minutes*
Equipment: *electric coffee grinder and electric food processor*
Yield: *Makes 8 bars*

How bad do you want to be? There is no justification for eating chocolate. But if you throw in some flaxseed, at least it's in good company. Another estrogenic snack bar with an abundance of omega-3s, this concoction is more like a confection—with an inner layer of tempting chocolate chips and walnuts.

½ cup frozen apple juice concentrate
2 cups pitted dates
1¼ cups flaxseed

3 tablespoons unsweetened cocoa powder
⅓ cup chocolate chips
⅓ cup chopped walnuts

1. Place the apple juice concentrate and dates in a saucepan. Cover and cook over medium-high heat for 5 minutes, until softened.

2. While the dates cook, grind the flaxseed in an electric coffee grinder ⅓ cup at a time. Pour the ground seeds into a food processor with the S blade inserted. Add the softened dried dates and cocoa powder.

3. Process until the mixture is doughlike. If the mixture rises above the processor blades, shut off the machine and push the mixture down with a spatula. Then, turn the machine back on. When the dough is fully mixed, it will form a ball in the well of the food processor.

4. Press half of the dough into a 9×9-inch nonstick pan. Sprinkle with chocolate chips and nuts. Press the remaining half of the dough over the chips and nuts. Cut into eight bars. (Make three evenly spaced cuts in one direction and one in the other.) Remove from the pan. Place in a storage container or in plastic sandwich bags. Refrigerate.

PLANT ESTROGEN ESTIMATE: 2½ PORTIONS PER BAR

PEANUT BUTTER-NUT BARS

Work and Cooking Time: *under 20 minutes*
Equipment: *electric coffee grinder and electric food processor*
Yield: *Makes 8 bars*

These peanut butter treats pack all of the estrogenic goodness and the heart-healthy omega-3 oils of the other snack bars. The peanut butter and soy nuts also make this one mighty high in protein, and the peanut butter makes the soy nuts taste more convincingly peanutlike.

½ cup frozen apple juice concentrate
2 cups dried apples or apricots
1¼ cups flaxseed

2½ tablespoons peanut butter
1 cup whole soy nuts
3 tablespoons chopped soy nuts

1. Place the apple juice concentrate and dried fruit in a saucepan. Cover and cook over medium-high heat for 5 minutes, until softened.

2. While the fruit cooks, grind the flaxseed in an electric coffee grinder ⅓ cup at a time. Pour the ground seeds into a food processor with the S blade inserted. Add the softened dried fruit and the peanut butter. Process until the mixture is doughlike. If the mixture rises above the processor blades, shut off the machine and push the mixture down with a spatula. Then, turn the machine back on. When the dough is fully mixed, it will form a ball in the well of the food processor. Turn the dough into a bowl. Mix in the whole soy nuts.

3. Sprinkle half of the chopped soy nuts over the bottom of a 9×9-inch nonstick pan. Press the dough into the pan. Sprinkle with remaining nuts. Cut into eight bars. (Make

three evenly spaced cuts in one direction and one in the other.) Remove from the pan. Place in a storage container or in plastic sandwich bags. Refrigerate.

CRISPY RICE BARS

Work and Cooking Time: *under 10 minutes*
Equipment: *electric coffee grinder*
Yield: *Makes 8 bars*

To me, these bars taste the way Rice Krispies bars should taste—crunchy and just a little gooey. But if you really still like marshmallow and margarine, these estrogenic treats might disappoint you.

There's a trick to getting the texture right; it's all in the timing. The rice syrup needs to boil for at least 1 full minute but not more than 2 minutes. If it boils for less than 1 minute, the rice cereal turns soggy. If it boils for more than 2 minutes, the bars get hard.

3 cups crispy brown-rice cereal
1 cup flaxseed

⅔ cup brown-rice syrup

1. Place the rice cereal in a medium-size mixing bowl. Grind the flaxseed in an electric coffee grinder ⅓ cup at a time . Add to the bowl.

2. Pour the rice syrup into a heavy-bottomed saucepan. Cook over medium-high heat. Boil for 1 minute. Place a spoon in the rice syrup. Slowly pour the syrup from the spoon. When the drip solidifies in midair, the syrup is ready to use. Pour it over the rice cereal and the ground flaxseed. Mix thoroughly.

3. Pour the mixture into a 9×9-inch nonstick or oiled pan. Refrigerate until cooled. Cut into eight bars. (Make three evenly spaced cuts in one direction and one in the other.) Remove from the pan. Place in a storage container or in plastic sandwich bags. Refrigerate.

PEANUT CRISPS

⚏

Work and Cooking Time: *under 10 minutes*
Equipment: *electric coffee grinder*
Yield: *Makes 8 bars*

Peanut brittle with an estrogenic inoculation! This treat, while not as sweet as candy, is high in protein and filled with heart-healthy omega-3 oils.

The texture of the treat will depend on how long the barley malt boils. If it boils for less than 1 minute, it will be sticky and shapeless. If it boils for 3 minutes, it will create a very hard brittle.

1 cup flaxseed
3 tablespoons peanut butter

2 cups soy nuts
½ cup barley malt

1. Grind the flaxseed in an electric coffee grinder ⅓ cup at a time. Pour into a bowl. Add the peanut butter. Mix with a wooden spoon until thoroughly combined. Stir in the soy nuts.

2. Pour the malt into a heavy-bottomed saucepan. Cook over medium-high heat. Allow the malt to boil for 1 minute. Pour into the bowl with the flaxseed, peanut butter, and soy nuts. Mix all of the ingredients completely.

3. Pour into a 9×9-inch nonstick or oiled pan. Allow to cool. Cut into eight bars. (Make three evenly spaced cuts in one direction and one in the other.) Remove from the pan. Place in a storage container or in plastic sandwich bags. Refrigerate.

PLANT ESTROGEN ESTIMATE: 2¾ PORTIONS PER BAR

CINNAMON-MOLASSES-NUT BARS

Work and Cooking Time: *under 10 minutes*
Equipment: *electric coffee grinder*
Yield: *Makes 8 bars*

Like a molasses brittle—and the blackstrap molasses and cinnamon in this treat increase its calcium content.

The trick to the texture is in the timing. If the barley malt and molasses boil for less than a minute, the nuts will never form a bar. If they boil for more than 3 minutes, you just might find the bar too brittle to bite.

1 cup flaxseed
1 tablespoon ground cinnamon
2 cups soy nuts

⅔ cup barley malt
2 tablespoons blackstrap molasses

1. Grind the flaxseed in an electric coffee grinder ⅓ cup at a time. Pour into a bowl. Add the cinnamon and soy nuts.

2. Pour the malt and molasses into a heavy-bottomed saucepan. Cook over medium-high heat. When the mixture has boiled for 1 minute, pour it over the flaxseed and soy nuts. Mix thoroughly.

3. Pour into a 9×9-inch nonstick or oiled pan. Allow to cool. Cut into eight bars. (Make three evenly spaced cuts in one direction and one in the other.) Remove from the pan. Place in a storage container or in plastic sandwich bags. Refrigerate.

> **PLANT ESTROGEN ESTIMATE: 2¾ PORTIONS PER BAR**

CRISPY CHOCOLATE BARS

≋

Work and Cooking Time: *under 10 minutes*
Equipment: *electric coffee grinder*
Yield: *Makes 8 bars*

I can't resist chocolate. But when I make these bars, at least I satisfy my urge in a low-fat, plant estrogen–packed form.

To keep the rice crisp, be sure to boil the barley malt for at least 1 minute. But don't boil it for too long; boiling for 3 minutes will turn your crispy bars into rock-candy crunch.

3 cups crispy brown-rice cereal	1 cup flaxseed
3 tablespoons unsweetened cocoa powder	¾ cup barley malt

1. Pour the rice cereal into a bowl. Add the cocoa powder. Grind the flaxseed in an electric coffee grinder ⅓ cup at a time. Pour over the cereal and cocoa.

2. Pour the malt into a heavy-bottomed saucepan. Cook over medium-high heat. Boil the malt for 1 minute. Pour over the flaxseed mixture. Mix thoroughly.

3. Press into a 9×9-inch nonstick or oiled pan. Allow to cool. Cut into eight bars. (Make three evenly spaced cuts in one direction and one in the other.) Remove from the pan. Place in a storage container or in plastic sandwich bags. Refrigerate.

PLANT ESTROGEN ESTIMATE: **2** PORTIONS PER BAR

≋ NUTTY SNACKS

It's hard to stop munching these nutty snacks, designed to be eaten by the handful. Throw them into a bowl and settle down to some guilt-free snacking. Or throw them into a plastic bag and take them along to munch at the movies, on a hike, or just on the run.

If munching on handfuls of crispy treats is your favorite way to eat estrogen, try the granola and cold-cereal recipes in the breakfast chapter. You can add more variety to your snacking with low-fat crunchy cereals.

CINNAMON APPLES AND MALTED NUTS

Work and Cooking Time: *under 10 minutes*
Baking Time: *4 minutes*
Equipment: *electric coffee grinder*
Yield: *Makes 4 servings*

Dried apples and nuts encased in a cinnamon-and-malt coating. This munchable mix not only gives you the estrogenic duo of flaxseed and soy, it also comes with a healthy measure of boron—a mineral that may benefit bones and elevate estrogen.

1 cup soy nuts

1 cup dried apples

1 teaspoon ground cinnamon

1 teaspoon grated orange rind

½ cup flaxseed

½ cup barley malt

1. Preheat the oven to 350°F.

2. Place the soy nuts, apples, cinnamon, and orange rind in a medium-size mixing bowl.

3. Grind the flaxseed in an electric coffee grinder. Add the ground seeds to the soy nuts and apples.

4. Pour the malt into a small saucepan. Cook over medium heat until it thins to a syrup. Add to the soy-nut mixture. Stir with a wooden spoon until all of the ingredients are combined and coated with malt.

5. Spread over a cookie sheet. Bake for 4 minutes, until the nuts are toasted. Remove from the oven. Using a spatula, loosen from the cookie sheet while still warm. Cool.

PLANT ESTROGEN ESTIMATE: 2¾ PORTIONS PER SERVING

MALTED POPCORN AND NUTS

Work and Cooking Time: *under 10 minutes*
Baking Time: *4 minutes*
Equipment: *electric coffee grinder*
Yield: *Makes 4 servings*

Not quite Cracker Jack, this not-so-sweet popcorn treat is healthy enough to eat for breakfast.

3 cups popped corn
1 cup soy nuts

½ cup flaxseed
⅔ cup barley malt

1. Preheat the oven to 350°F.

2. Place the popcorn and soy nuts in a medium-size mixing bowl.

3. Grind the flaxseed in an electric coffee grinder. Add the ground seeds to the popcorn and soy nuts.

4. Pour the malt into a small saucepan. Cook over medium heat until it thins to a syrup. Add to the popcorn and nuts. Stir with a wooden spoon until all of the ingredients are combined and coated with malt.

5. Spread over a cookie sheet. Bake for 4 minutes, until the nuts are toasted. Remove from the oven. Using a spatula, loosen from the cookie sheet while still warm. Cool.

PLANT ESTROGEN ESTIMATE: 2¾ PORTIONS PER SERVING

SWEET CURRIED NUTS

Work and Cooking Time: *under 10 minutes*
Baking Time: *4 minutes*
Equipment: *electric coffee grinder*
Yield: *Makes 4 servings*

Sweet and savory, this snack makes for a crunchy change of pace.

1 cup soy nuts
⅔ cup raisins
1 tablespoon curry powder

1 teaspoon ground cinnamon
⅓ cup flaxseed
½ cup barley malt

1. Preheat the oven to 350°F.

2. Place the soy nuts, raisins, curry powder, and cinnamon in a medium-size mixing bowl.

3. Grind the flaxseed in an electric coffee grinder. Add the ground seeds to the soy nut–raisin mixture.

4. Pour the malt into a small saucepan. Cook over medium heat until it thins to a syrup. Add to the soy nuts and raisins. Stir with a wooden spoon until all of the ingredients are combined and coated with malt.

5. Spread over a cookie sheet. Bake for 4 minutes, until the nuts are toasted. Remove from the oven. Using a spatula, loosen from the cookie sheet while still warm. Cool.

> **PLANT ESTROGEN ESTIMATE: 2¾ PORTIONS PER SERVING**

TRAIL MIX

Work and Cooking Time: *under 10 minutes*
Baking Time: *15 minutes*
Equipment: *electric coffee grinder*
Yield: *Makes 6 servings*

Lots of soy nuts. Lots of flaxseed. Lots of dried fruit. Lots of estrogenic energy in every bite.

2 cups soy nuts	⅔ cup raisins
1 cup flaxseed	⅔ cup chopped dried apricots
½ cup barley malt	⅔ cup dried cranberries or chopped dates

1. Preheat the oven to 300°F.

2. Place the soy nuts in a medium-size mixing bowl. Grind the flaxseed in an electric coffee grinder ⅓ cup at a time. Pour into the mixing bowl.

3. Pour the malt into a small saucepan. Cook over high heat. Boil for 3 minutes. Add to the soy nuts and seeds. Stir with a wooden spoon until all of the ingredients are combined and coated with malt.

4. Spread over a cookie sheet. Bake for 15 minutes, until the nuts are toasted. Remove from the oven. Using a spatula, loosen from the cookie sheet while still warm. Mix in the dried fruit. Cool. Store in the refrigerator.

PLANT ESTROGEN ESTIMATE: 3⅔ PORTIONS PER SERVING

PUFFED CORN BALL TRAIL MIX

Work and Cooking Time: *under 10 minutes*
Baking Time: *15 minutes*
Equipment: *electric coffee grinder*
Yield: *Makes 6 servings*

When Manju, my older daughter, was at college, we brought her rations—granola with puffed corn. She complained, "I love the puffed corn balls, but my roommate eats them; she picks them out of the cereal." If you love the puffed corn balls in this trail mix, feel free to pick them out. They're coated with flaxseed, so you'll get a goodly dose of estrogenic goodness.

3 cups puffed corn cereal

2 cups soy nuts

1 cup flaxseed

1 cup brown-rice syrup

⅔ cup dried fruit (optional)

1. Preheat the oven to 300°F.

2. Place the corn cereal and soy nuts in a medium-size mixing bowl. Grind the flaxseed in an electric coffee grinder ⅓ cup at a time. Pour into the mixing bowl.

3. Pour the rice syrup into a small saucepan. Cook over high heat. Boil for 3 minutes. Add to the cereal, nuts, and seeds. Stir with a wooden spoon until all of the ingredients are combined and coated with syrup.

4. Spread over a cookie sheet. Bake for 15 minutes, until the nuts are toasted. Remove from the oven. Using a spatula, loosen from the cookie sheet while still warm. If desired, mix in the dried fruit. Cool. Store in the refrigerator.

PLANT ESTROGEN ESTIMATE: 3⅔ PORTIONS PER SERVING

MAPLE NUTS

Work and Cooking Time: *under 5 minutes*
Baking Time: *12 minutes*
Yield: *Makes 4 servings*

Soy nuts tend to be dry. Just tossing them with a little maple syrup and baking them gives them a sweet, lightly crispy coating.

2 cups soy nuts
¼ cup maple syrup

1. Preheat the oven to 300°F.

2. Place the soy nuts in a mixing bowl. Stir in the maple syrup to coat the nuts evenly.

3. Spread over a cookie sheet. Bake for 12 minutes, until the nuts are lightly toasted. Remove from the oven. Using a spatula, loosen from the cookie sheet while still warm. Cool. Store in the refrigerator.

PLANT ESTROGEN ESTIMATE: 1½ PORTIONS PER SERVING

VARIATION: *Mix in 1 teaspoon of your favorite spice—such as cinnamon or cardamom—before baking.*

HOT MUGS AND SUPER THERMOSES

If you're like me, a coffee mug travels with you everywhere. In quest of oral gratification, I sip continually. My habit hasn't totally changed with this "change" in my life. I still keep a cup in hand constantly, but the coffee's gone . . . well, almost gone. I love coffee. The taste, the high, the ritual—I confess, I'm addicted. I crave it. One cappuccino and I want a double. I look for any excuse to drink it. But I know the rap on coffee. It leaches calcium. I feel its badness in my bones. If I drink one cup of coffee a day for three days in a row and stop, I get a massive headache. If I keep drinking the stuff, my night sweats return. But I'm learning. Instead of filling up on high-octane coffee, I nearly always imbibe estrogenically inoculated hot drinks.

The switch from cappuccino to liquid soybeans can be made only by following one essential commandment—*add more flavor.* Cartons of soy milk labeled "chocolate" or "vanilla" don't taste like chocolate or vanilla. They taste like . . . *soy.* These flavorings just don't convert the taste of soy into a drinkable delight. Cardamom, nutmeg, or almond extract does.

SIMPLY SPICED MUGFULS

Work and Cooking Time: *under 5 minutes*
Yield: *Makes 2 servings*

This is my basic coffee substitute. I drink it whenever I want—at work, in my car, in the kitchen, on the couch. For me, sipping from a soy-filled mug is a sign of liberation. My mug has a logo that says, "I'm a grown-up. I don't have to put my mug down for anyone!"

2 cups soy milk (plain, vanilla, or chocolate)
1 teaspoon ground cardamom or nutmeg

Heat the soy milk. Stir in the spice. Taste. If needed, add more spice.

PLANT ESTROGEN ESTIMATE: **1** PORTION PER SERVING

QUICK ALMOND MILK

Work and Cooking Time: *under 5 minutes*
Yield: *Makes 2 servings*

I like to think of this simple hot drink as Italian *orzata*—that delightful steamed milk–and–almond delicacy. It's not, of course, but it is a tasty way to keep a giant-size mug by my side.

Here's more good news: If you have a cappuccino maker, soy milk steams up well. With a frothy top, almond milk does become as satisfying as *orzata*.

2 cups soy milk
½ teaspoon almond extract

Heat the soy milk. Stir in the almond extract. Taste. If needed, add more almond extract.

PLANT ESTROGEN ESTIMATE: 1 PORTION PER SERVING

ALMOST COFFEE BY THE MUG

Work and Cooking Time: *under 5 minutes*
Yield: *Makes 1 serving*

It's not coffee! But it is good, easy, quick, healthy, and phytoestrogen-filled.

Grain coffees like Cafix, Postum, or Pero don't cover the taste of soy any better than small quantities of chocolate or vanilla. To really make a hot grain-coffee drink tasty, you need to add more flavoring.

You can, of course, bring grain coffee to a whole other level of enjoyment by steaming it. Soy milk bubbles and froths better than most any milk—certainly better than skim milk.

1 cup soy milk

1 teaspoon grain coffee

½ teaspoon ground cardamom or nutmeg, or almond extract

Heat the soy milk. Dissolve the grain coffee in the hot milk. Stir in the spice or flavoring.

PLANT ESTROGEN ESTIMATE: 1 PORTION PER SERVING

SPICED HOT MILK BY THE QUART

Work and Cooking Time: *under 5 minutes*
Yield: *Makes 4 servings*

Like your daily hot drinks by the thermos? Want to serve a simple hot after-dinner "tea"? Making spiced hot milk by the quart is nearly as quick as making it by the mugful.

1 quart soy milk (vanilla or chocolate)

1 tablespoon ground cardamom, cinnamon, or nutmeg

Pour the soy milk into a heavy-bottomed saucepan. Stir in the ground spice and cook over medium-high heat until the milk begins to bubble. Pour into a thermos or serving carafe.

PLANT ESTROGEN ESTIMATE: 1 PORTION PER SERVING

EAST INDIAN-STYLE SPICED MILK OR TEA

Work and Cooking Time: *10 to 15 minutes*
Yield: *Makes 4 servings*

In terms of taste, the tea in this recipe is optional. But if you need an occasional caffeine fix, take comfort: Reports have it that Japanese green tea has heart-healthy, anti-aging effects. The only problem is—it's green. If drinking a milky green liquid seems just too weird, try to find Japanese *roasted* green tea—it's brown.

If you don't have cinnamon sticks, forget the cinnamon in this recipe. Ground cinnamon tends to settle to the bottom and get slimy.

The longer this hot concoction simmers, the stronger its spicy flavor.

1 quart soy milk
6 ⅛×1-inch slices fresh ginger
1 teaspoon ground cardamom
¼ teaspoon ground nutmeg

4 cinnamon sticks
4 teabags of Japanese roasted green tea
 (optional)

Pour the milk into a heavy-bottomed saucepan. Add the remaining ingredients. Simmer over medium-high heat for 10 to 15 minutes. Pour into a thermos or serving carafe.

PLANT ESTROGEN ESTIMATE: **1** PORTION PER SERVING

DELICIOUS AND FESTIVE SHAKES

Milk shakes and frappes—ice-cream temptation in a soda glass tastes so satisfying. But after the enjoyment, there's a price to pay: That heavy, bloated feeling sets in. Within two hours, the fat literally sticks to the insides of the arteries.

Want to indulge without the aftereffect? Do I have a treat for you! Try these estrogenic shakes. Every single frothy serving of these festive shakes delivers more than a single portion of plant estrogens. The secret is the silken tofu—it adds thickness and creaminess. So, drink to your heart's delight. No artery-clogging cream. No cholesterol. In fact, these high-protein, estrogen-rich shakes will do your heart good!

FESTIVE NOG

Work Time: *under 5 minutes*
Equipment: *electric blender*
Yield: *Makes 4 servings*

A great holiday recipe, this nog whips up frothy enough to serve on any festive occasion—like breakfast!

It will maintain its frothy bubbles for at least two hours in the refrigerator.

3 cups cold soy milk

1 cake (19 ounces) silken tofu

1 teaspoon ground nutmeg

2 teaspoons ground cinnamon

2 teaspoons anise extract

1 tablespoon vanilla extract

3 tablespoons maple syrup

Place all of the ingredients in an electric blender. Start the blender on low speed and turn it up to high. Blend for a minimum of 5 minutes, until frothy. Taste. If needed, add more flavoring. Serve immediately or chill before serving.

PLANT ESTROGEN ESTIMATE: 1¾ PORTIONS PER SERVING

ORANGE SHAKE

Work Time: *under 5 minutes*
Equipment: *electric blender*
Yield: *Makes 1 serving*

Sara, my teenage daughter, says, "You could give this to little kids. They'd like it."

Orange juice easily overcomes the taste of soy. The result—a high-C, highly estrogenic indulgence even a kid could love.

¼ cup frozen orange juice concentrate
½ cake (9½ ounces) silken tofu

⅓ cup soy milk
2 teaspoons vanilla extract

Place all of the ingredients in an electric blender. Blend until smooth and frothy. Taste. If needed, add more flavoring. Serve.

PLANT ESTROGEN ESTIMATE: 2⅓ PORTIONS PER SERVING

CINNAMON-COFFEE SHAKE

Work Time: *under 5 minutes*
Equipment: *electric blender*
Yield: *Makes 1 serving*

My husband walked in the room. I said, "Drink this." He sipped and commented, "It's good, but it's not really coffee." If you like grain coffee—Cafix, Pero, or Postum—you'll like this shake just fine. But if you're an espresso connoisseur, expect to be disappointed.

1 tablespoon grain coffee
½ cake (9½ ounces) silken tofu
⅓ cup soy milk

1 teaspoon ground cinnamon
½ teaspoon blackstrap molasses
1 tablespoon maple syrup

Place all of the ingredients in an electric blender. Blend until smooth and frothy. Taste. If needed, add more flavoring. Scrve.

PLANT ESTROGEN ESTIMATE: 2⅓ PORTIONS PER SERVING

ALMOND SHAKE

Work Time: *under 5 minutes*
Equipment: *electric blender*
Yield: *Makes 1 serving*

Almond extract does a fine job of subjugating the taste of soy!

½ cake (9½ ounces) silken tofu
⅔ cup soy milk
½ teaspoon almond extract

2 teaspoons vanilla extract
2 tablespoons maple syrup

Place all of the ingredients in an electric blender. Blend until smooth and frothy. Taste. If needed, add more flavoring. Serve.

PLANT ESTROGEN ESTIMATE: 2⅔ PORTIONS PER SERVING

GINGER SHAKE

Work Time: *under 5 minutes*
Equipment: *electric blender*
Yield: *Makes 1 serving*

1½ tablespoons chopped fresh ginger
½ cake (9½ ounces) silken tofu
¾ cup soy milk

1 tablespoon maple syrup
1 teaspoon vanilla extract

Place all of the ingredients in an electric blender. Blend until smooth, creamy, and bubbly. Taste. If needed, add more flavoring. Serve.

PLANT ESTROGEN ESTIMATE: 2¾ PORTIONS PER SERVING

CHOCOLATE SHAKE

Work Time: *under 5 minutes*
Equipment: *electric blender*
Yield: *Makes 1 serving*

When nothing but chocolate will do, this is a great indulgence.

2 tablespoons unsweetened cocoa powder
½ cake (9½ ounces) silken tofu
¾ cup soy milk

2 tablespoons maple syrup
1 teaspoon blackstrap molasses
2 teaspoons vanilla extract

Place all of the ingredients in an electric blender. Blend until smooth and frothy. Taste. If needed, add more flavoring. Serve.

PLANT ESTROGEN ESTIMATE: 2¾ PORTIONS PER SERVING

PEPPERMINT SHAKE

Work Time: *under 5 minutes*
Equipment: *electric blender*
Yield: *Makes 1 serving*

For my good friend Phillip, sipping a cold peppermint shake relieves stress. I just had to include a recipe.

¼ teaspoon peppermint extract
¼ cake (4¾ ounces) silken tofu
1 cup soy milk

1 tablespoon honey
2 teaspoons vanilla extract

Place all of the ingredients in an electric blender. Blend until smooth and frothy. Taste. If needed, add more flavoring. Serve.

PLANT ESTROGEN ESTIMATE: 1¼ PORTIONS PER SERVING

CHERRY FROSTY SHAKE

Work Time: *under 5 minutes*
Equipment: *electric blender*
Yield: *Makes 1 serving*

Using frozen pitted cherries makes this shake a frozen delight.

1 cup frozen pitted cherries
¾ cup soy milk
¼ cake (4¾ ounces) silken tofu

1½ tablespoons all-fruit cherry jam
1 teaspoon lemon extract

Place all of the ingredients in an electric blender. Blend until smooth and frothy. Taste. If needed, add more flavoring. Serve.

PLANT ESTROGEN ESTIMATE: 1¼ PORTIONS PER SERVING

STRAWBERRY FROSTY FRAPPE

Work Time: *under 5 minutes*
Equipment: *electric blender*
Yield: *Makes 1 serving*

The perfect summertime fruit frappe—thick and icy. You won't miss ice cream for a minute.

1 cup frozen strawberries
½ cake (9½ ounces) silken tofu
¾ cup soy milk

2 teaspoons all-fruit strawberry jam
1 teaspoon orange extract

Place all of the ingredients in an electric blender. Blend until smooth and frothy. Taste. If needed, add more flavoring. Serve.

PLANT ESTROGEN ESTIMATE: 2¾ PORTIONS PER SERVING

CHOCOLATE FROSTY FRAPPE

Work Time: *under 5 minutes*
Equipment: *electric blender*
Yield: *Makes 1 serving*

It's chocolate. How can it be bad? Well, chocolate is a caffeine source! So drink this one in moderation.

½ cup soy milk
¼ cake (4¾ ounces) silken tofu
2 tablespoons unsweetened cocoa powder

2 tablespoons maple syrup
1 teaspoon blackstrap molasses
8 ice cubes

Place all of the ingredients in an electric blender. Blend until the ice cubes are chopped and the shake is creamy. Taste. If needed, add more flavoring. Serve.

PLANT ESTROGEN ESTIMATE: 1½ PORTIONS PER SERVING

BANANA FROSTY SHAKE

Work Time: *under 5 minutes*
Equipment: *electric blender*
Yield: *Makes 1 serving*

Frozen melon balls thicken and sweeten this icy banana shake.

1 banana
½ cake (9½ ounces) silken tofu
1 teaspoon banana extract
¼ cup soy milk

1 tablespoon maple syrup
2 tablespoons lemon juice
1 cup frozen melon balls

Place all of the ingredients in an electric blender. Blend until the frozen melon balls are chopped and the shake is creamy. Taste. If needed, add more flavoring. Serve.

PLANT ESTROGEN ESTIMATE: 2¼ PORTIONS PER SERVING

ORANGE FRAPPE

Work Time: *under 5 minutes*
Equipment: *electric blender*
Yield: *Makes 1 serving*

Orange is one of those special flavors that cover the taste of tofu easily. This creamy, cool, hot-day drink is nothing but good for you.

¼ cake (4¾ ounces) silken tofu
½ cup soy milk
3 tablespoons frozen orange juice concentrate
1 teaspoon vanilla extract

1 teaspoon orange extract
2 tablespoons maple syrup
8 ice cubes

Place all of the ingredients in an electric blender. Blend until the ice cubes are chopped and the shake is creamy. Taste. If needed, add more flavoring. Serve.

PLANT ESTROGEN ESTIMATE: 1¼ PORTIONS PER SERVING

Four

Breakfast

Forget the eggs. Forgo the butter. Forsake the cholesterol. Wake up to an estrogenic feast. Pancakes, cereals, omelets, scrambles, and crêpes are on the morning menu!

The Clark Kents of superfoods, soy and flaxseed, look like humble fodder. In fact, at this very moment, some chickens somewhere are feeding on flaxseed. Their creative keepers noticed that the infusion of flaxseed lowers chicken cholesterol. They hope for a new invention and the resurgence of the perfect food—the low-cholesterol egg! But the clandestine cook in the menopausal kitchen doesn't need their invention. Who needs low-cholesterol eggs when you can make no-cholesterol, cholesterol-lowering morning meals? Who needs a flax-modified egg when you can simply use the flax instead of the egg? Who needs scrambled eggs when you can scramble a heart-healthy alternative? Are you skeptical? Do you doubt that within these humble seeds and beans lies the power to make a thoroughly satisfying breakfast? If you can banish your disbelief, you might be surprised.

Usually you have two choices in granola—fat-filled or low-fat. The fat-filled stuff is crunchy. The low-fat stuff is soggy. These cold cereals are different. They're crisp without added oil. The crunch comes from maple, malt, or rice syrup. These sweeteners are great! They're healthier than most. But best of all, when you heat them, they harden. They coat cereal with crunch. They help make megaportions of plant estrogen and omega-3 essential fatty acids part of a simple wake-up meal.

MAPLE-NUT CRUNCH

Work Time: *under 5 minutes*
Baking Time: *10 minutes*
Equipment: *electric coffee grinder*
Yield: *Makes 2 servings*

To infuse your morning with mighty portions of plant estrogen, eat this cold cereal with soy milk. To boost the estrogenic effect with added boron, just add dried fruit. Or use this cereal like sugar: Sprinkle it generously on hot cereals and make yourself an estrogenic meal.

If you make this recipe, keep plenty on hand. At our house, we're always finding new ways to use it. I sprinkle it on fruit salad. Michael eats it directly from the bowl. And Brenda, my daughter's roommate, dips strawberries in it.

To vary this recipe, add a tablespoon of ground orange peel, cardamom, cinnamon, or nutmeg.

1 cup flaxseed
⅓ cup maple syrup
¼ cup chopped walnuts

1. Preheat the oven to 300°F.

2. Grind the flaxseed in an electric coffee grinder ⅓ cup at a time. Place the ground seeds in a bowl.

3. Add the maple syrup and walnuts. Stir until the seeds are thoroughly coated with maple syrup.

4. Spread the mixture over a cookie sheet. Bake for 5 minutes. Stir. Bake for 5 more minutes, until lightly toasted. Immediately loosen from the cookie sheet with a spatula. Cool. Serve with soy milk. Store any unused portion in the refrigerator.

PLANT ESTROGEN ESTIMATE: 8 PORTIONS PER SERVING

MALTED CINNAMON CRUNCH

Work and Cooking Time: *under 5 minutes*
Baking Time: *10 minutes*
Equipment: *electric coffee grinder*
Yield: *Makes 2 servings*

A serving of plant estrogen in every bite. Eat a bowl of this malted flaxseed crunch and you've consumed a full course of protective plant estrogens in just one sitting. When the day calls for steaming hot cereal, this can double as sugar. Sprinkle it on without restraint. At our house, we all eat it like candy.

1 cup flaxseed
⅓ cup barley malt
2 teaspoons ground cinnamon

1. Preheat the oven to 350°F.

2. Grind the flaxseed in an electric coffee grinder ⅓ cup at a time. Place the ground seeds in a bowl.

3. Pour the malt into a small saucepan. Bring to a boil. Allow to boil for 1 minute. Pour the hot malt over the ground seeds and add the cinnamon. Stir until the malt coats the seeds evenly.

4. Spread the mixture over a cookie sheet. Bake for 10 minutes, until lightly toasted. Immediately loosen from the cookie sheet with a spatula. Cool. Serve with soy milk. Store any unused portion in the refrigerator.

PLANT ESTROGEN ESTIMATE: **8** PORTIONS PER SERVING

DATE-NUT GRANOLA

Work and Cooking Time: *under 10 minutes*
Baking Time: *15 minutes*
Equipment: *electric coffee grinder*
Yield: *Makes 4 servings*

If you love crunch, you have crunch! Eat it for breakfast or for a snack. Enjoy it with soy milk or by the handful.

1 cup rolled oats
1 cup flaxseed
½ cup chopped dates
½ cup chopped almonds

2 tablespoons ground cinnamon
⅔ cup barley malt
1 teaspoon vanilla extract

1. Preheat the oven to 350°F.
2. Place the oats in a bowl. Grind ¾ cup of the flaxseed in an electric coffee grinder in two batches. Add to the oats. Add the remaining whole flaxseed, dates, almonds, and cinnamon.
3. Pour the malt into a small saucepan. Bring to a gentle boil. Stir in the vanilla. Allow to boil for 1 minute. Pour over the oat-and-flaxseed mixture. Stir, coating the oats and flaxseed completely with hot malt.
4. Spread the mixture over a cookie sheet. Bake for 15 minutes, stirring every 5 minutes. Remove from the oven when lightly toasted. Immediately loosen from the cookie sheet with a spatula. Cool. Serve with soy milk. Store any unused portion in the refrigerator.

PLANT ESTROGEN ESTIMATE: **4** PORTIONS PER SERVING

CINNAMON-MALT GRANOLA

Work and Cooking Time: *under 10 minutes*
Baking Time: *10 minutes*
Equipment: *electric coffee grinder*
Yield: *Makes 4 servings*

Look at those plant estrogen estimates! It's unbelievable how much comes packed in a bowl filled with this crunchy cereal and soy milk. If morning cereal is not your cup of tea, just snack on this granola at teatime.

1 cup flaxseed

1 cup rolled oats

¾ cup soy nuts

1 teaspoon ground cinnamon

½ cup barley malt

½ cup raisins

1. Preheat the oven to 350°F.

2. Grind ½ cup of the flaxseed in an electric coffee grinder. Pour it into a bowl. Add the remaining whole flaxseed, oats, soy nuts, and cinnamon.

3. Pour the malt into a small saucepan. Bring to a gentle boil. Allow to boil for 1 minute. Pour over the oat-and-flaxseed mixture. Stir, coating the oats and flaxseed completely with hot malt.

4. Spread the mixture over a cookie sheet. Bake for 10 minutes, stirring after 5 minutes. Remove from the oven when lightly toasted. Immediately loosen from the cookie sheet with a spatula. Mix in the raisins. Cool. Serve with soy milk. Store any unused portion in the refrigerator.

PLANT ESTROGEN ESTIMATE: 4 PORTIONS PER SERVING

NEW ENGLAND MAPLE-CRANBERRY GRANOLA

Work and Cooking Time: *under 10 minutes*
Baking Time: *10 minutes*
Equipment: *electric coffee grinder*
Yield: *Makes 4 servings*

From the day I was born until I went off to college, I lived on the same neighborly street in a small New England town. I still live in New England. I wouldn't have it any other way. This is a breakfast treat from home, filled with all the plant estrogen you could ever want in one bowl. I love to munch on it any time of day.

½ cup plus ⅓ cup flaxseed
1 cup rolled oats
⅓ cup rice syrup

3 tablespoons maple syrup
⅓ cup chopped walnuts
⅔ cup dried cranberries

1. Preheat the oven to 350°F.
2. Grind ½ cup of flaxseed in an electric coffee grinder. Pour it into a bowl. Add the remaining whole flaxseed and the oats.
3. Pour the rice syrup into a small saucepan. Bring to a gentle boil. Allow to boil for 1 minute. Stir in the maple syrup. Pour over the oat-and-flaxseed mixture. Stir, coating the oats and flaxseed completely with hot syrup.
4. Spread the mixture over a cookie sheet. Bake for 10 minutes, stirring after 5 minutes. Remove from the oven when lightly toasted. Immediately loosen from the cookie sheet with a spatula. Mix in the walnuts and cranberries. Cool. Serve with soy milk. Store any unused portion in the refrigerator.

PLANT ESTROGEN ESTIMATE: 4 PORTIONS PER SERVING

≋ HOT CEREALS

If you love a hot-and-hearty porridge in the morning, these three tips will transform your basic breakfast into an estrogenic meal:

TIP 1: Spoon Maple-Nut Crunch, Malted Cinnamon Crunch, or Simple Cereal Sprinkle on your hot cereal.

TIP 2: Cook your cereal with soy milk instead of water.

TIP 3: Stir in dried fruit—chopped prunes, peaches, apricots, dates, or raisins.

These minor alterations really improve the taste. The Sprinkles taste like crunchy brown sugar. The soy milk adds a creamy richness. The dried fruit adds still more flavor. The combination is a high-protein meal laden with heart-protective omega-3s and laced with plenty of plant estrogens and estrogen-friendly boron.

Here's another bit of advice: If you're tempted to up your estrogen count by stirring ground flaxseed into your hot cereal, do so at your own risk. A little ground flaxseed makes the cereal slippery. A lot of ground flaxseed transforms hot cereal into a gooey gob. Some people actually like the texture. You might. My husband, Michael, does. He eats his cereal slightly slimy every day.

SIMPLE CEREAL SPRINKLE

Work Time: *under 5 minutes*
Equipment: *electric coffee grinder*
Yield: *Makes 1¼ cups*

Spoon this simple combination on top of your cereal, and it will add a slightly nutty taste. Stir it in, and it will give any cereal the gooey feel of oatmeal.

½ cup flaxseed
½ cup raw sugar

Grind the flaxseed in an electric coffee grinder. Place it in a small serving bowl. Add the sugar. Stir. Place in a sugar bowl. Store in the refrigerator between servings.

PLANT ESTROGEN ESTIMATE: ⅓ PORTION PER TABLESPOON

CREAMED RICE CEREAL

Work and Cooking Time: *10 minutes*
Yield: *Makes 1 serving*

This light and creamy cereal has three unappealing secrets: flour, soy milk, and miso. These ingredients might cause even the most dedicated hot-cereal eater to skip this one. Don't. Try it—it's really good.

⅓ cup brown-rice flour
1¾ cups soy milk
1 teaspoon yellow miso (optional)

1 teaspoon vanilla extract
2 tablespoons dried fruit (optional)

1. Place the flour and soy milk in a heavy-bottomed saucepan. Cook over medium-high heat, stirring occasionally, until the mixture begins to thicken.

2. Reduce the heat to medium and add the miso, if desired. Stir constantly until the mixture is fully thickened. Remove from the heat.

3. Stir in the vanilla, and add the dried fruit, if desired. Serve.

PLANT ESTROGEN ESTIMATE: 1¾ PORTIONS PER SERVING

CREAMED WHEAT CEREAL

Work and Cooking Time: *under 10 minutes*
Yield: *Makes 1 serving*

When I realized how creamed wheat cereal is usually made, I was appalled: It's coarse white flour cooked in water. It's thick gravy without the flavoring. Now that you know, don't be scared off. If you liked creamed wheat before you knew, you'll really enjoy this simple whole-wheat estrogenic version.

⅓ cup whole-wheat flour

2 cups soy milk

1 teaspoon yellow miso (optional)

1 teaspoon ground cinnamon or cardamom

1 teaspoon maple syrup

2 tablespoons chopped dried fruit (optional)

1. Whisk the whole-wheat flour into ½ cup of the soy milk until dissolved.

2. Heat the remaining 1½ cups of soy milk in a heavy-bottomed saucepan over medium-high heat. When it begins to boil, stir in the dissolved flour.

3. Reduce the heat. Add the miso, if desired, spice, and maple syrup. Stir constantly until thickened. Stir in the dried fruit, if desired. Serve.

> PLANT ESTROGEN ESTIMATE: **2** PORTIONS PER SERVING

CRACKED-WHEAT CEREAL

Work and Cooking Time: *40 minutes*

Yield: *Makes 1 serving*

Making cracked-wheat cereal is time-consuming. But if you like a crunchy, creamy, whole-grain cereal, it's worth the wait.

⅓ cup cracked wheat

1 cup soy milk

1 teaspoon ground cinnamon

¼ cup raisins

1. Place the cracked wheat and ⅔ cup of water in a heavy-bottomed saucepan. Boil for 10 minutes.

2. Add the soy milk and cinnamon. Reduce the heat to low.

3. Cook for 30 minutes, until the cereal is creamy. Stir in the raisins. Serve.

> PLANT ESTROGEN ESTIMATE: **1** PORTION PER SERVING

BROWN-RICE CEREAL

Work and Cooking Time: *1 hour*
Yield: *Makes 4 servings*

To make this cereal in the morning, you need leftover rice and time. If you have them, this hot cereal is almost as much fun to eat as rice pudding.

2 cups cooked brown rice

2 cups soy milk

2 teaspoons ground cardamom

¼ cup chopped dried fruit (optional)

Place all of the ingredients except the dried fruit in a heavy-bottomed saucepan. Simmer, stirring occasionally, for 1 hour. If desired, stir in the dried fruit 15 minutes before removing from the heat. Serve.

PLANT ESTROGEN ESTIMATE: ½ PORTION PER SERVING

CREAMY CARDAMOM OATMEAL

Work and Cooking Time: *under 20 minutes*
Yield: *Makes 1 serving*

This easy-to-cook oatmeal is an everyday staple with a flavorful twist and a creamy texture.

2 cups soy milk

⅔ cup rolled oats

½ teaspoon ground cardamom

3 tablespoons chopped dried dates or apricots (optional)

1. Pour the soy milk into a saucepan. Bring to a boil. Stir in the oats and cardamom.
2. Reduce the heat to medium-low. Simmer for 15 minutes. Stir in the dried fruit, if desired.

PLANT ESTROGEN ESTIMATE: 2 PORTIONS PER SERVING

≋ PANCAKES

Estrogenic pancakes require a bit of care and understanding. Like all pancakes, they need to be ladled onto a preheated, lightly oiled or non-stick heavy frying pan or griddle. Cook these pancakes over medium heat (not high heat). You need patience. Wait until they have bubbles all over the surface. When the batter looks slightly darker and just a bit dried out, flip them. If the pan has been heated to the right temperature, they will be brown—not burned. Wait until the second side is brown. Serve. If you've waited long enough, the pancakes will be perfect. If you haven't, they'll be gooey inside.

LEMON-BLUEBERRY PANCAKES

≋

Work and Cooking Time: *under 20 minutes*
Equipment: *electric blender*
Yield: *Makes 2 generous servings*

Do your blueberries bleed? Do your pancakes come out purple? Does the extra blueberry juice invade the batter, making it too liquid? Mine did. Then I learned not to add the blueberries to the batter. Dust the blueberries with flour and put them on the pancakes as they cook. The juice will stay where it belongs—inside the blueberries.

1½ cups plus 1 tablespoon unbleached white flour

1 teaspoon baking soda

1 teaspoon baking powder

1½ teaspoons grated lemon rind

2 cups soy milk

1 teaspoon yellow miso

2 tablespoons lemon juice

2 tablespoons frozen apple juice concentrate

⅓ cup flaxseed

1 cup fresh or frozen blueberries

1. Heat a nonstick or oiled griddle or frying pan over medium heat.

2. Place the 1½ cups of flour, baking soda, baking powder, and lemon rind in a medium-size mixing bowl. Stir until well combined.

3. Place the soy milk, miso, lemon juice, apple juice concentrate, and flaxseed in an electric blender. Blend until the seeds disintegrate and the mixture bubbles. Pour the liquid mixture into the dry ingredients. Stir until combined.

4. Place the blueberries in a small bowl. Add the tablespoon of flour. Toss, coating the blueberries.

5. Ladle the batter onto the preheated griddle or frying pan. Spoon a few blueberries onto each pancake as it cooks. Allow to cook until the surface bubbles and appears less liquid. Flip. Cook until lightly browned. Serve.

PLANT ESTROGEN ESTIMATE: **4** PORTIONS PER SERVING

SWEDISH OATMEAL PANCAKES

Work and Cooking Time: *under 20 minutes*
Equipment: *electric coffee grinder*
Yield: *Makes 2 generous servings*

The lightest pancakes of all!

⅓ cup flaxseed
1 cup whole-wheat pastry flour
1 cup rolled oats

1 tablespoon baking powder
3 cups soy milk
2 tablespoons frozen apple juice concentrate

1. Heat a nonstick or oiled griddle or frying pan over medium heat.

2. Grind the flaxseed in an electric coffee grinder. Pour into a medium-size mixing bowl. Add the flour, oats, and baking powder. Stir until well combined. Add the soy milk and apple juice concentrate. Mix with a wire whisk.

3. Ladle the batter onto the preheated griddle or frying pan. Allow to cook until the surface bubbles and appears less liquid. Flip. Cook until lightly browned. Serve.

PLANT ESTROGEN ESTIMATE: **4** PORTIONS PER SERVING

BUCKWHEAT PANCAKES

Work and Cooking Time: *under 20 minutes*
Equipment: *electric blender*
Yield: *Makes 2 generous servings*

If you like buckwheat, these pancake will please you. If you don't care for buckwheat's hearty, distinctive taste, don't even try them.

¾ cup buckwheat flour
¼ cup unbleached white flour
1½ teaspoons baking powder
1 teaspoon baking soda
1 teaspoon ground cinnamon

1 tablespoon lemon juice
1 tablespoon maple syrup
2 cups soy milk
¼ cup flaxseed
Blueberries dusted with flour (optional)

1. Heat a nonstick or oiled griddle or frying pan over medium heat.

2. Place the buckwheat flour, white flour, baking powder, baking soda, and cinnamon in a medium-size mixing bowl. Stir until well combined.

3. Place the lemon juice, maple syrup, soy milk, and flaxseed in an electric blender. Blend until the seeds disintegrate and the mixture bubbles. Pour the liquid mixture into the dry ingredients. Stir until combined.

4. Ladle the batter onto the preheated griddle or frying pan. Spoon a few blueberries onto each pancake as it cooks, if desired. Allow to cook until the surface bubbles and appears less liquid. Flip. Cook until lightly browned. Serve.

PLANT ESTROGEN ESTIMATE: 3 PORTIONS PER SERVING

RICE-WHEAT PANCAKES

Work and Cooking Time: *under 20 minutes*
Equipment: *electric blender*
Yield: *Makes 2 servings*

Basic pancakes for any day!

¾ cup brown-rice flour
¾ cup whole-wheat pastry flour
1 teaspoon baking soda
2 teaspoons baking powder
1 teaspoon vanilla extract

1 tablespoon maple syrup
2 tablespoons lemon juice
1 tablespoon yellow miso
2 cups soy milk
⅓ cup flaxseed

1. Heat a nonstick or oiled griddle or frying pan over medium heat.

2. Place the rice flour, wheat flour, baking soda, and baking powder in a medium-size mixing bowl. Stir until well combined.

3. Place the remaining ingredients in an electric blender. Blend until the seeds disintegrate and the mixture bubbles. Pour the liquid mixture into the dry ingredients. Stir until combined.

4. Ladle the batter onto the preheated griddle or frying pan. Allow to cook until the surface bubbles and appears less liquid. Flip. Cook until lightly browned. Serve.

PLANT ESTROGEN ESTIMATE: **4** PORTIONS PER SERVING

APPLE-ORANGE PANCAKES

Work and Cooking Time: *under 20 minutes*
Equipment: *electric blender*
Yield: *Makes 2 generous servings*

A very tasty pancake treat!

1½ cups unbleached flour

1 teaspoon baking soda

2 teaspoons baking powder

½ teaspoon grated orange rind

2 tablespoons frozen orange juice concentrate

1 teaspoon yellow miso

2 cups soy milk

⅓ cup flaxseed

1 apple, grated

1. Heat a nonstick or oiled griddle or frying pan over medium heat.

2. Place the flour, baking soda, baking powder, and orange rind in a medium-size mixing bowl. Stir until well combined.

3. Place the orange juice concentrate, miso, soy milk, and flaxseed in an electric blender. Blend until the seeds disintegrate and the mixture bubbles. Pour the liquid mixture into the dry ingredients. Add the apple. Stir until combined.

4. Ladle the batter onto the preheated griddle or frying pan. Allow to cook until the surface bubbles and appears less liquid. Flip. Cook until lightly browned. Serve.

PLANT ESTROGEN ESTIMATE: **4** PORTIONS PER SERVING

≋ PANCAKE SYRUPS

At least half the pleasure of eating pancakes is the syrup. These syrups are estrogenic delights. The light, creamy syrups blend silken tofu and soy milk with maple syrup, all-fruit preserves, or frozen juice concentrates. The focus on concentrated fruits—preserves, jams, and juice concentrates—brings more than just the pleasure of their taste. Fruit tends to be high in boron, a mineral that may help to boost estrogen levels and benefit bones. Concentrated forms of fruit give higher concentrations of boron. So pour on the syrup!

CREAMY FRUITY SYRUP

⊛

Work Time: *under 5 minutes*
Equipment: *electric blender*
Yield: *Makes about 1 cup*

Always lightly creamy, this syrup can take on any fruity flavor you wish. Just choose your jam. Cherry, strawberry, peach, apricot, blueberry—each will bring its own flavor to this basic, versatile recipe.

½ cake (9½ ounces) silken tofu
½ cup soy milk
⅔ cup all-fruit jam

1 teaspoon lemon extract
1 teaspoon vanilla extract

Place all of the ingredients in an electric blender. Blend until smooth. Taste. If needed, add more flavoring. Serve with pancakes or French toast.

PLANT ESTROGEN ESTIMATE: ABOUT ⅓ PORTION PER **2**-TABLESPOON SERVING

CREAMY ORANGE SYRUP

⊛

Work Time: *under 5 minutes*
Equipment: *electric blender*
Yield: *Makes 1 cup*

Orange goes so well with apple. Pour this syrup over apple pancakes.

½ cake (9½ ounces) silken tofu
½ cup soy milk
2 tablespoons frozen orange juice concentrate

2 tablespoons frozen apple juice concentrate
¼ cup all-fruit orange marmalade
1 teaspoon orange extract

Place all of the ingredients in an electric blender. Blend until smooth. Taste. If needed, add more flavoring. Serve with pancakes.

PLANT ESTROGEN ESTIMATE: ¾ PORTION PER ¼-CUP SERVING

MAPLE-ALMOND CREAMY SYRUP

Work Time: *under 5 minutes*
Equipment: *electric blender*
Yield: *Makes about 1¼ cups*

½ cake (9½ ounces) silken tofu
½ cup soy milk
½ cup maple syrup

2 teaspoons vanilla extract
1 teaspoon almond extract
3 tablespoons chopped almonds

This syrup heightens the flavor of any pancake!

Place the tofu, soy milk, maple syrup, vanilla extract, and almond extract in an electric blender. Blend until smooth. Taste. If needed, add more flavoring. Pour into a serving bowl. Stir in the nuts. Serve with pancakes.

PLANT ESTROGEN ESTIMATE: ½ PORTION PER ¼-CUP SERVING

MOLASSES CREAM SYRUP

Work Time: *under 5 minutes*
Equipment: *electric blender*
Yield: *Makes 1¼ cups*

Molasses hikes the calcium content! Pour this syrup liberally over your favorite pancakes or spoon it over hot cereal.

½ cake (9½ ounces) silken tofu
½ cup soy milk

½ cup table molasses
1 tablespoon blackstrap molasses

Place all of the ingredients in an electric blender. Blend until smooth.

MAPLE-NUT SYRUP

Work Time: *under 5 minutes*
Yield: *Makes 1 cup*

This thick, only lightly creamy, nut-filled syrup is a bit fancier than the usual.

½ cup maple syrup
1 teaspoon vanilla extract

½ cup soy milk
2 tablespoons chopped walnuts

Whisk the ingredients together. The mixture will thicken in about 5 minutes. Serve with pancakes.

SWEET CRÊPES OR BLINTZES

Tofu is amazing stuff! I love crêpes. I tried and tried to make crêpes from tofu. I failed and failed. Desperate, I mixed some jam and vanilla with firm tofu. I couldn't imagine that it would work. The batter didn't pour. It spread like frosting. So I frosted the bottom of a nonstick cake pan, leaving a slightly thicker lip around the edge of the crêpe, not letting the batter touch the edge of the pan. Impatient, I baked it at 500°F. I waited 8 to 10 minutes. The rim of the crêpe turned brown.

The middle gelled. It worked! I could fold it. I could fill it. I had made a high-protein, low-fat, estrogenic crêpe!

Now, with tofu, I don't make one crêpe at a time. I bake them in every nonstick 9-inch cake pan I own. If I run out of cake pans, I grab pie plates.

BASIC CRÊPES

Work Time: *under 10 minutes*
Baking Time: *8 to 10 minutes*
Equipment: *electric food processor*
Yield: *Makes 2 servings of 2 crêpes*

Basic crêpes work well with just a little syrup.

1 cake (16 ounces) firm tofu
1 tablespoon vanilla extract

2 tablespoons maple syrup

1. Preheat the oven to 500°F.

2. Place all of the ingredients in a food processor with the S blade inserted. Process for 2 minutes, until smooth and silky.

3. Spoon the mixture into the center of four nonstick or oiled 9-inch round cake pans, dividing the mixture evenly. Using the back of a soup spoon, carefully spread the tofu mixture, making expanding circles and gradually moving the mixture toward the edge of the pans. Do not allow the mixture to touch the edge of the cake pans. Distribute the batter as evenly as possible, leaving the outer edge of the batter slightly thicker than the middle. This will prevent uneven cooking or spotty burning.

4. Bake for 8 to 10 minutes, until the edges of the crêpes are brown, the batter has a crêpelike texture, and the crêpes can be folded without breaking.

5. While still in the cake pans, gently fold the crêpes in half and then in quarters. Using a spatula, move the folded crêpes to a serving plate. Serve with any syrup.

PLANT ESTROGEN ESTIMATE: **2** PORTIONS PER SERVING

CHERRY-FILLED CRÊPES WITH
CREAMY CHERRY SAUCE

Work and Cooking Time: *under 25 minutes*
Baking Time: *8 to 10 minutes*
Equipment: *electric food processor*
Yield: *Makes 2 serving of 2 crêpes*

Want a fancy brunch food? Or a delightful feast for high tea? This sweet combination of crêpes, cherry filling, and creamy cherry sauce is the answer. It brings a fancy flair to your table, along with a megadose of plant estrogens.

Crêpes
1 cake (16 ounces) firm tofu
1 tablespoon vanilla extract
2 tablespoons maple syrup

Filling and Topping
16 ounces frozen pitted cherries, thawed, with juice
1 tablespoon cornstarch
2 tablespoons frozen apple juice concentrate
1½ teaspoons almond extract
½ cake (9½ ounces) silken tofu
½ cup all-fruit cherry preserves

1. Preheat the oven to 500°F.

2. Place all of the crêpe ingredients in a food processor with the S blade inserted. Process for 2 minutes, until smooth and silky.

3. Spoon the crêpe mixture into the center of four nonstick or oiled 9-inch round cake pans, dividing the mixture evenly. Using the back of a soup spoon, carefully spread the tofu mixture, making expanding circles and gradually moving the mixture toward the edge of the pans. Do not allow the mixture to touch the edge of the cake pans. Distribute the batter as evenly as possible, leaving the outer edge of the batter slightly thicker than the middle. This will prevent uneven cooking or spotty burning. Bake for 8 to 10 minutes, until the edges of the crêpes are brown, the batter has a crêpelike texture, and the crêpes can be folded without breaking. While still in the cake pans, gently fold the crêpes in half and then in quarters. Using a spatula, move the folded crêpes to serving plates.

4. While the crêpes bake, prepare the filling and topping: Cook the cherries over medium-high heat. Dissolve the cornstarch in the apple juice concentrate. When the

cherries and their juice are simmering, stir in the dissolved cornstarch. Continue stirring until the mixture has thickened. Remove from the heat. Add the almond extract.

5. To make the creamy topping, place ¼ cup of the prepared cherry filling in the food processor. Add the silken tofu and cherry preserves. Process until smooth and silky.

6. Unfold the crêpes. Spoon a quarter of the cherry filling down the center of each crêpe. Fold the sides over the filling. Top with creamy cherry sauce. Serve.

PLANT ESTROGEN ESTIMATE: 2¼ PORTIONS PER SERVING

STRAWBERRY CRÊPES

Work Time: *under 25 minutes*
Baking Time: *8 to 10 minutes*
Equipment: *electric food processor*
Yield: *Makes 2 servings of 2 crêpes*

Thoroughly festive strawberry crêpes! Strawberry juice concentrate gives the topping a bright pink color. If you can't find it, any juice concentrate will do.

Crêpes
1 cake (16 ounces) firm tofu
2 tablespoons all-fruit strawberry jam

Filling
¼ cake (4¾ ounces) silken tofu
2 tablespoons all-fruit strawberry jam
1 teaspoon lemon extract
1 pint strawberries, chopped

Topping
½ cake (9½ ounces) silken tofu
2 tablespoons all-fruit strawberry jam
1 teaspoon lemon extract
⅓ cup frozen strawberry or apple juice
    concentrate

1. Preheat the oven to 500°F.

2. Place all of the crêpe ingredients in a food processor with the S blade inserted. Process for 2 minutes, until smooth and silky.

3. Spoon the crêpe mixture into the center of four nonstick or oiled 9-inch round cake pans, dividing the mixture evenly. Using the back of a soup spoon, carefully spread the tofu mixture, making expanding circles and gradually moving the mixture toward the edge of the pans. Do not allow the mixture to touch the edge of the cake pans. Distribute the batter as evenly as possible, leaving the outer edge of the batter slightly thicker than the middle. This will prevent uneven cooking or spotty burning. Bake for 8 to 10 minutes, until the edges of the crêpes are brown, the batter has a crêpelike texture, and the crêpes can be folded without breaking. While still in the cake pans, gently fold the crêpes in half and then in quarters. Using a spatula, move the folded crêpes to serving plates.

4. While the crêpes bake, prepare the filling and topping: To make the filling, place the tofu, jam, and lemon extract in the food processor. Process until smooth. Taste. If needed, add more flavoring. Turn into a small mixing bowl. Stir in the strawberries.

5. To make the topping, place the tofu, jam, lemon extract, and juice concentrate in the food processor. Process until smooth and silky. Pour into a serving bowl.

6. Unfold the crêpes. Spoon a quarter of the filling down the center of each crêpe. Fold the sides over the filling. Top with creamy sauce. Serve.

PLANT ESTROGEN ESTIMATE: 3½ PORTIONS PER SERVING

APPLE-ORANGE BLINTZES

Work Time: *under 25 minutes*
Baking Time: *8 to 10 minutes*
Equipment: *electric food processor*
Yield: *Makes 2 servings of 2 blintzes*

As near as I can tell, the only difference between crêpes and blintzes is how they are folded: The ends of a blintz are folded over the filling, making a complete little package.

Blintzes

1 cake (16 ounces) firm tofu
1 tablespoon vanilla extract
2 tablespoons maple syrup

Filling

½ cake (8 ounces) soft tofu
2 tablespoons all-fruit orange marmalade
1 tablespoon ground cinnamon
1 tablespoon grated orange rind
1 teaspoon orange extract
2 apples, grated

Topping

½ cup orange juice
½ cup frozen apple juice concentrate
1 teaspoon orange extract
¼ cake (4½ ounces) silken tofu

1. Preheat the oven to 500°F.

2. Place all of the blintz ingredients in a food processor with the S blade inserted. Process for 2 minutes, until smooth and silky.

3. Spoon the blintz mixture into the center of four nonstick or oiled 9-inch round cake pans, dividing the mixture evenly. Using the back of a soup spoon, carefully spread the tofu mixture, making expanding circles and gradually moving the mixture toward the edge of the pans. Do not allow the mixture to touch the edge of the cake pans. Distribute the batter as evenly as possible, leaving the outer edge of the batter slightly thicker than the middle. This will prevent uneven cooking or spotty burning. Bake for 8 to 10 minutes, until the edges are brown, the batter has a crêpelike texture, and the blintzes can be folded without breaking. While still in the cake pans, gently fold the blintzes in half and then in quarters. Using a spatula, move the folded blintzes to serving plates.

4. While the blintzes bake, prepare the filling and topping: To make the filling, place the soft tofu, marmalade, cinnamon, orange rind, and orange extract in the food processor. Process until smooth. Turn into a small mixing bowl. Stir in the grated apple.

5. To make the topping, place the juice, juice concentrate, orange extract, and silken tofu in the food processor. Process until smooth and creamy. Pour into a serving bowl.

6. Unfold the blintzes. Spoon a quarter of the apple filling into the center of each blintz. Fold two sides partially over the filling. Fold the other two sides completely over the filling, forming a rectangular package. Top with creamy sauce. Serve.

PLANT ESTROGEN ESTIMATE: **3½ PORTIONS PER SERVING**

PEACH-PECAN BLINTZES

Work Time: *under 25 minutes*
Baking Time: *8 to 10 minutes*
Equipment: *electric food processor*
Yield: *Makes 2 servings of 2 blintzes*

Another perfect blintz with a creamy, crunchy filling.

Blintzes
1 cake (16 ounces) firm tofu
2 tablespoons all-fruit peach preserves
½ teaspoon almond extract

Filling
½ cake (8 ounces) soft tofu
2 tablespoons all-fruit peach preserves
1 teaspoon almond extract
1 peach, chopped
2 tablespoons chopped pecans

Topping
1 cup frozen white grape juice concentrate
1 tablespoon all-fruit peach preserves
2 teaspoons vanilla extract
¼ cake silken tofu

1. Preheat the oven to 500°F.

2. Place all of the blintz ingredients in a food processor with the S blade inserted. Process for 2 minutes, until smooth and silky.

3. Spoon the blintz mixture into the center of four nonstick or oiled 9-inch round cake pans, dividing the mixture evenly. Using the back of a soup spoon, carefully spread the tofu mixture, making expanding circles and gradually moving the mixture toward the edge of the pans. Do not allow the mixture to touch the edge of the pans. Distribute the batter as evenly as possible, leaving the outer edge of the batter slightly thicker than the middle. This will prevent uneven cooking or spotty burning. Bake for 8 to 10 minutes, until the edges are brown, the batter has a crêpelike texture, and the blintzes can be folded without breaking. While still in the cake pans, gently fold the blintzes in half and then in quarters. Using a spatula, move the folded blintzes to serving plates.

4. While the blintzes bake, prepare the filling and topping: To make the filling, place the soft tofu, preserves, and almond extract in the food processor. Process until smooth. Turn into a small mixing bowl. Stir in the peach and nuts.

5. To make the topping, place the juice concentrate, preserves, vanilla, and silken tofu in the food processor. Process until smooth and creamy. Pour into a serving bowl.

6. Unfold the blintzes. Spoon a quarter of the peach filling into the center of each blintz. Fold two sides partially over the filling. Fold the other two sides completely over the filling, forming a rectangular package. Top with creamy sauce. Serve.

PLANT ESTROGEN ESTIMATE: 3½ PORTIONS PER SERVING

〰 SCRAMBLES

A little turmeric for color, a little garlic for flavor, a little salt for taste, then mash and scramble. I think I've invented the perfect egg taste-alike. I say, "Doesn't this taste just like eggs!" In unison, my daughters exclaim, "No!" Manju voices her opinion: "It's good. It tastes kind of like eggs. People will like it." Sara chimes in, "Some people might think it's eggs. They look like eggs." Manju adds, "If you don't tell people, they might actually think it's eggs. The way you make it—scrambled— what else could they be?" My children are right. They keep me honest.

I won't lie to you. I won't tell you that tofu scrambled magically turns into egg. If you're an egg lover, estrogenic scrambles might not make it. But if you're motivated, if you want a cholesterol-cutting, estrogen-enriching alternative, you may love these scrambles.

GARLIC-AND-ONION SCRAMBLE

Work and Cooking Time: *under 10 minutes*
Yield: *Makes 1 serving*

This easy, flavorful scramble provides a simple, cholesterol-lowering, estrogen-imparting breakfast. Make it with soft tofu if you like your scramble soft. Choose firm tofu if you like your scramble firm.

This recipe makes one hearty serving. To make a meal for more people, just multiply by the number of servings you need.

Spray oil	½ cake (8 ounces) soft or firm tofu
1 garlic clove, minced	⅛ teaspoon turmeric
½ small onion, chopped	Salt and pepper

1. Spray a heavy frying pan with oil and place over medium-high heat. Sauté the garlic and onion.

2. Mash the tofu with a fork or potato masher. Mash in the turmeric. Sprinkle lightly with salt and pepper. Add the tofu to the browned onion and garlic. Cook, stirring occasionally, until fully heated. Serve.

PLANT ESTROGEN ESTIMATE: **2** PORTIONS PER SERVING

SALSA-AND-SAUSAGE SCRAMBLE

Work and Cooking Time: *under 10 minutes*
Yield: *Makes 1 serving*

Add soy sausage and salsa to a basic scramble to make a hearty, high-protein, estrogen-packed meal.

To make your scramble soft, use soft tofu. To make it firm, use firm tofu. This one-serving recipe can be multiplied to serve as many people as you like with a minimum of extra time and effort.

Spray oil
1 garlic clove, minced
½ small onion, chopped
3 soy sausages, sliced
½ cake (8 ounces) soft or firm tofu

⅛ teaspoon turmeric
Salt and pepper
½ tomato, chopped
2 tablespoons salsa

1. Spray a heavy frying pan with oil and place over medium-high heat. Sauté the garlic and onion. Add the sausage.

2. While the garlic, onion, and sausage cook, mash the tofu with a fork or potato masher. Mash in the turmeric. Sprinkle lightly with salt and pepper. Add the tofu to the browned garlic, onion, and sausage. Stir in the chopped tomato and salsa. Cook, stirring occasionally, just until heated. Serve.

PLANT ESTROGEN ESTIMATE: 2½ PORTIONS PER SERVING

MACKEREL SCRAMBLE

Work and Cooking Time: *under 10 minutes*
Yield: *Makes 2 servings*

If you adore the flavor of smoked fish, you'll love this wonderful combination.

1 onion, chopped
2 garlic cloves, sliced
1 cake (19 ounces) silken tofu

¼ teaspoon turmeric
4 ounces smoked mackerel

1. Heat a nonstick or lightly oiled frying pan over medium-high heat. Sauté the onion and garlic until the onion is browned.

2. Mash the tofu and turmeric together in a mixing bowl. Cut the mackerel into small pieces and add to the tofu. Add the tofu mixture to the browned onion and garlic. Cook, stirring occasionally, just until heated. Serve.

PLANT ESTROGEN ESTIMATE: **2** PORTIONS PER SERVING

VEGGIE SCRAMBLE

Work and Cooking Time: *under 10 minutes*
Yield: *Makes 1 serving*

A basic scramble with your favorite vegetables—how can it be bad? You can substitute any vegetable that suits your fancy. For a family breakfast or a party brunch, multiply the recipe.

Spray oil
1 garlic clove, minced
½ small onion, chopped
¼ cup chopped mushrooms
¼ cup chopped broccoli

¼ cup chopped green or red bell pepper
½ cake silken, soft, or firm tofu
⅛ teaspoon turmeric
Salt and pepper

1. Spray a heavy frying pan with oil and place over medium-high heat. Sauté the garlic, onion, and mushrooms. Add the broccoli. When the broccoli can be pierced with a fork, add the bell pepper.

2. Mash the tofu with a fork or potato masher. Mash in the turmeric. Sprinkle lightly with salt and pepper. Add the tofu to the vegetables. Cook, stirring occasionally, just until heated. Serve.

PLANT ESTROGEN ESTIMATE: **2** PORTIONS PER SERVING

OMELETS

Tofu omelets work best with lots of wonderful fillings and even some flavorful toppings. The omelet itself looks and tastes surprisingly egg-like, but it's not an identical twin.

Here are the basics of tofu omelet making:

- Use *firm* tofu: Softer tofu takes forever to bake and comes out rubbery.
- Bake in a cake pan: When fried in a frying pan, puréed tofu never turns into an omelet—it burns on the bottom and stays soft on top.
- Spread the batter like frosting over the bottom of the cake pan and leave a thick lip around the outer rim to prevent burning.
- Leave a space between the edge of the pan and the rim of the tofu to make the omelet easy to remove.
- Bake at 500°F. Tofu breaks when folded if cooked at lower temperatures.
- Bake for 12 minutes, until just firm enough to fold. Baked too long, the omelet will be rubbery. Baked for too short a time, it will be mushy.
- Stuff with your favorite omelet fillings and top with your best-loved toppings. These additions are the best part!

BASIC OMELET

⠿

Work and Baking Time: *under 20 minutes*
Equipment: *electric food processor*
Yield: *Makes 1 omelet*

1 garlic clove, quartered

½ cake (8 ounces) firm tofu

⅛ teaspoon turmeric

1 teaspoon Dijon mustard

Salt

Any favorite filling and topping

1. Preheat the oven to 500°F.

2. Place all of the ingredients (except the filling and topping) in a food processor with the S blade inserted and blend until smooth.

3. Pour the mixture into the center of a 9-inch nonstick cake pan. Using the back of a soup spoon, carefully spread the tofu mixture, making expanding circles and gradually moving the mixture toward the edge of the pan. Bake for 12 minutes, until the underside of the omelet is lightly browned and the top has gelled.

4. While the omelet bakes, prepare the filling and topping.

5. Remove the omelet from the oven. Fold it in half. Move it to a serving plate. Unfold. Spoon the filling over half the omelet. Fold the other half over the filling. Spoon on the topping. Serve.

PLANT ESTROGEN ESTIMATE: **2** PORTIONS PER SERVING

WILD-MUSHROOM OMELET

⠿

Work and Baking Time: *under 20 minutes*
Equipment: *electric food processor*
Yield: *Makes 1 omelet*

With a tasty filling of wild mushrooms, this omelet makes cutting cholesterol and increasing estrogen a morning delight.

Since this omelet is made in the oven in a cake pan, it's easy to make two, three, or even four at a time. Just multiply the recipe and use more cake pans.

Omelet	**Filling**
1 garlic clove, quartered	Spray oil
½ cake (8 ounces) firm tofu	2 cups chopped fresh wild mushrooms (porto-
⅛ teaspoon turmeric	bello, shiitake, and/or oyster)
1 teaspoon light-brown barley-soybean miso	2 garlic cloves, minced
	1 teaspoon dark soybean miso

1. Preheat the oven to 500°F.

2. Place the garlic, tofu, turmeric, and miso in a food processor with the S blade inserted and blend until smooth and silky.

3. Pour the mixture into the center of a 9-inch nonstick cake pan. Using the back of a soup spoon, carefully spread the tofu mixture, making expanding circles and gradually moving the mixture toward the edge of the pan. Bake for 12 minutes, until the underside of the omelet is lightly browned and the top has gelled.

4. While the omelet bakes, prepare the mushroom filling: Spray a frying pan with oil and place over medium-high heat. Sauté the mushrooms and garlic. Dissolve the miso in 1 tablespoon of water. Add. Continue to sauté until the mushrooms are browned. If the mushrooms stick to the frying pan, add another tablespoon of water. Reduce the heat to low.

5. Remove the omelet from the oven. Fold it in half. Move it to a serving plate. Unfold. Spoon the mushroom mixture over half the omelet. Fold the other half over the sautéed mushrooms. Serve.

PLANT ESTROGEN ESTIMATE: **2** PORTIONS PER OMELET

MEXICAN OMELET

Work and Baking Time: *under 20 minutes*
Equipment: *electric food processor*
Yield: *Makes 1 omelet*

Another omelet without eggs! The Mexican filling and topping make a hardy, choles-terol-cutting, estrogen-increasing wake-up meal.

Making the omelet in the oven means you can easily multiply the ingredients and have several omelets cooking at the same time.

Omelet	Filling
1 garlic clove, quartered	Spray oil
½ cake (8 ounces) firm tofu	1 garlic clove, minced
⅛ teaspoon turmeric	½ onion, chopped
1 teaspoon dried cilantro or 1 tablespoon chopped fresh cilantro	½ red bell pepper, chopped
	½ green bell pepper, chopped
1 teaspoon light-brown barley-soybean miso	½ avocado, peeled and sliced
	Salsa

1. Preheat the oven to 500°F.

2. Place all of the omelet ingredients in a food processor with the S blade inserted and blend until smooth.

3. Pour the mixture into the center of a 9-inch nonstick cake pan. Using the back of a soup spoon, carefully spread the tofu mixture, making expanding circles and gradually moving the mixture toward the edge of the pan. Bake for 12 minutes, until the under-side of the omelet is lightly browned and the top has gelled.

4. While the omelet bakes, prepare the filling: Spray a frying pan with oil and place over medium-high heat. Sauté the garlic and onion until lightly browned. Add the bell pepper. Remove from the heat and stir in the sliced avocado.

5. Remove the omelet from the oven. Fold it in half. Move it to a serving plate. Unfold. Spoon the filling over half the omelet. Fold the other half over the filling. Top with salsa before serving.

PLANT ESTROGEN ESTIMATE: **2** PORTIONS PER SERVING

SPINACH-AND-BACIN OMELET

Work and Baking Time: *under 20 minutes*
Equipment: *electric food processor*
Yield: *Makes 1 omelet*

Spinach gives this omelet a healthy portion of calcium. The bacin bits are actually little bits of soy protein colored with beets. They can be found in the spice section of most natural foods stores and in many supermarkets.

Omelet
1 garlic clove, quartered
½ cake (8 ounces) firm tofu
⅛ teaspoon turmeric
1 teaspoon Dijon mustard
Salt

Filling
Spray oil
1 garlic clove, minced
½ onion, chopped
6 ounces fresh spinach
1 tablespoon bacin bits

1. Preheat the oven to 500°F.

2. Place all of the omelet ingredients in a food processor with the S blade inserted and blend until smooth.

3. Pour the mixture into the center of a 9-inch nonstick cake pan. Using the back of a soup spoon, carefully spread the tofu mixture, making expanding circles and gradually moving the mixture toward the edge of the pan. Bake for 12 minutes, until the underside of the omelet is lightly browned and the top has gelled.

4. While the omelet bakes, prepare the filling: Spray a frying pan with oil and place over medium-high heat. Sauté the garlic and onion until brown. Add the spinach. Cook until limp. Stir in the bacin bits.

5. Remove the omelet from the oven. Fold it in half. Move it to a serving plate. Unfold. Spoon the filling over half the omelet. Fold the other half over the filling. Serve.

PLANT ESTROGEN ESTIMATE: **2** PORTIONS PER SERVING

Five

Spreads and Breads

Everybody's a bread eater. Some munch away on a simple slice. Others spread that bread with something sweet, salty, spicy, or fishy. Most people buy their bread, but some actually make their own. Some prefer muffins to bread. Some like a sweet bread. Some love to dunk crackers into a bowl of dip. So what's the point? Why am I writing this little essay on bread? I want you to know that however you eat your bread, there are recipes for you in this chapter. There are spreads, dips, and pâtés. There are crackers, muffins, and quick breads. And if you can't resist getting your hands in some dough . . . knead away—there are even yeast breads. Each and every bread recipe delivers estrogenic goodness. Along with your daily bread, you'll get your daily flaxseed or soy.

≋ BASIC SANDWICH SPREADS

What's a sandwich without mayonnaise and mustard? Ugh! What's a sandwich *with* mayonnaise and mustard? Many, many artery-clogging

calories. How do you get a yummy sandwich while you lower cholesterol and reduce calories? Make these estrogenic sandwich spreads.

ALL-PURPOSE MAYONNAISE

Work Time: *under 5 minutes*
Equipment: *electric food processor*
Yield: *Makes about 1 cup*

If you love mayonnaise, you'll be thrilled to have this recipe. Eat it without guilt—it's low
in calories and cholesterol-free. I spoon it onto every sandwich I eat.

2 garlic cloves, quartered
½ cake (8 ounces) soft tofu
1 tablespoon Dijon mustard

1 teaspoon apple cider vinegar
Salt

   Place the garlic in a food processor with the S blade inserted. Process until minced.
Add the tofu, mustard, and vinegar to the processor. Process until smooth. Add salt to
taste and process to mix in. Taste. If needed, add more mustard and salt. Place in a jar
and refrigerate.

PLANT ESTROGEN ESTIMATE: **2** PORTIONS PER RECIPE

CURRIED MAYONNAISE

Work Time: *under 5 minutes*
Equipment: *electric food processor*
Yield: *Makes 1 cup*

This curried version of mayonnaise has a slightly sweet flavor that is particularly tasty with chicken or turkey.

2 garlic cloves, quartered
½ cake (8 ounces) soft tofu
1 tablespoon apple cider vinegar

½ teaspoon ground cinnamon
1 tablespoon honey
1 tablespoon yellow miso

Place all of the ingredients in a food processor with the S blade inserted. Process for 4 minutes, until smooth and silky. Spoon into a jar and refrigerate. Spread generously on sandwiches.

PLANT ESTROGEN ESTIMATE: **2** PORTIONS PER RECIPE

PESTO SPREAD

Work Time: *under 10 minutes*
Equipment: *electric food processor*
Yield: *Makes 1½ cups*

This creamy tofu-based pesto provides a rich feel with less fat, more protein, and, naturally, a good bit of estrogen.

2 garlic cloves, quartered
2 cups firmly packed fresh basil leaves
½ cake (8 ounces) soft tofu

¼ cup walnuts or pine nuts
Salt

Place the garlic in a food processor with the S blade inserted. Mince. Add the basil leaves. Mince. Add the tofu and nuts. Process until smooth. Salt to taste. Serve as a dip for crackers or a spread for bread.

ROASTED GARLIC SPREAD

Work Time: *under 5 minutes*
Equipment: *electric food processor*
Yield: *Makes 1 cup*

This is a garlic lover's delight. Spread it on your favorite sandwich, or serve it with warm bread. It makes a great accompaniment to any meal.

To make this spread in a jiffy, you need bottled roasted garlic. I find it in the condiment section, near the mustard, in my supermarket.

1 cup bottled roasted garlic, drained
½ cake (8 ounces) soft tofu

2 tablespoons light-brown miso

Place all of the ingredients in a food processor with the S blade inserted. Process until smooth. Spoon into a jar and refrigerate. Use as a spread for bread.

PÂTÉS AND DIPS

Pâtés and dips are usually gourmet indulgences, but these versions aren't too rich for your health. Try them with bread, crackers, or cut-up vegetables—they'll give you only goodness.

GUACAMOLE

Work Time: *under 5 minutes*
Equipment: *electric food processor*
Yield: *Makes 1 cup*

This creamy version of the avocado-based favorite works well as a dip for chips or a topping on any Mexican dish.

2 garlic cloves, quartered
1 tablespoon fresh cilantro
¼ cake (4¾ ounces) silken tofu

1 avocado, peeled and quartered
1 teaspoon lemon juice
Salt

Place the garlic in a food processor with the S blade inserted. Mince. Add the cilantro. Mince. Add the tofu, avocado, and lemon juice. Process until smooth. Salt to taste. Serve.

PLANT ESTROGEN ESTIMATE: 1 PORTION PER RECIPE

HUMMUS

Work Time: *under 5 minutes*
Equipment: *electric food processor*
Yield: *Makes 1½ cups*

The flavor of tahini comes through strongly in this quickly concocted tofu hummus.

3 garlic cloves, quartered
½ cake (8 ounces) soft tofu
⅓ cup tahini

1 tablespoon lemon juice
2 tablespoons unsweetened soy milk
Salt

Place the garlic in a food processor with the S blade inserted. Mince. Add the remaining ingredients except salt. Process until smooth. Salt to taste. Serve.

PLANT ESTROGEN ESTIMATE: **2** PORTIONS PER RECIPE

ROASTED RED PEPPER–AND–GARLIC PÂTÉ

Work Time: *under 5 minutes*
Equipment: *electric food processor*
Yield: *Makes about 1 cup*

A tasty, bright-red pâté that works equally well as a spread for bread or a dip for chips or vegetables.

3 garlic cloves, quartered
7-ounce jar roasted red peppers

¼ cake (4 ounces) soft tofu

Place the garlic in a food processor with the S blade inserted. Mince. Drain the liquid from the red peppers. Add them to the food processor, along with the tofu. Purée until smooth.

PLANT ESTROGEN ESTIMATE: **1** PORTION PER RECIPE

BLUEFISH PÂTÉ

≋

Work and Cooking Time: *under 10 minutes*
Equipment: *electric food processor*
Yield: *Makes 1 cup*

Spoon this pâté on a pretty plate and surround it with melba toast or crackers. Guests will swear you bought it at the deli. When you say you made it, they'll think it's packed with high-calorie cream cheese. It's not!

It's low in calories and healthy enough to save for yourself. Spoon it on a baguette for a simply elegant lunch.

Spray oil

8 ounces bluefish fillet

¼ cake (4 ounces) firm tofu

2 teaspoons tamari

1 teaspoon Dijon mustard

1. Preheat the broiler.

2. Spray the bluefish lightly with oil. Broil for 3 minutes on each side, until cooked through.

3. Place the broiled fish in a food processor with the S blade inserted. Add the remaining ingredients. Process until smooth. Place on a serving plate or in a container.

PLANT ESTROGEN ESTIMATE: 1 PORTION PER RECIPE

SHIITAKE MUSHROOM PÂTÉ

Work Time: *under 5 minutes*
Waiting Time: *2 hours*
Equipment: *electric food processor*
Yield: *Makes about 1 cup*

This pâté captures the shiitake taste and increases its benefits with the addition of estrogenic soy. In natural foods stores and supermarkets, dried shiitake mushrooms are an expensive delicacy. In Chinese markets in large cities, they can be bought by the pound for a song. They keep forever, so buy in bulk.

Dried shiitakes require rehydrating. Cover them with warm water and let them sit for 2 hours. The mushrooms become chewy—almost oysterlike. Soaked in water and stored in the refrigerator, they'll keep for a week.

¾ cup dried shiitake mushrooms
2 garlic cloves, quartered

¼ cake (4 ounces) firm tofu
2 tablespoons tamari

1. Cover the mushrooms with warm water and let them sit for 2 hours, or until fully rehydrated.

2. Place the garlic in a food processor with the S blade inserted. Mince. Squeeze the water out of the rehydrated mushrooms and place them in the food processor with 3 tablespoons of the soaking water. Add the tofu and tamari and process until a pâté forms. Serve with bread or crackers.

> **PLANT ESTROGEN ESTIMATE: 1 PORTION PER RECIPE**

ARTICHOKE DIP

Work Time: *under 10 minutes*
Equipment: *electric food processor*
Yield: *Makes about 1½ cups*

A fun snack or an elegant appetizer, this dip goes especially well with whole-grain crackers.

3 garlic cloves, quartered
3 tablespoons lemon juice
½ cake (8 ounces) soft tofu
1 tablespoon tamari

8½-ounce can artichoke hearts, packed in
    water, drained
2 tablespoons small capers

Place the garlic in a food processor with the S blade inserted. Mince. Add the lemon juice, tofu, and tamari. Process until smooth. Add the artichokes. Process repeatedly, using the pulse setting, until the artichokes are finely chopped but not puréed. Turn into a bowl. Stir in the capers. Serve.

PLANT ESTROGEN ESTIMATE: **2** PORTIONS PER RECIPE

SMOKED MACKEREL PÂTÉ

Work Time: *under 5 minutes*
Equipment: *electric food processor*
Yield: *Makes ¾ cup*

The easiest pâté ever!

4 ounces smoked mackerel
¼ cake (4 ounces) soft tofu

Place the ingredients in a food processor with the S blade inserted. Process until smooth. Serve with crackers, bread, or bagels.

PLANT ESTROGEN ESTIMATE: 1 PORTION PER SERVING

≋ CRACKERS

Let's be honest. I don't know anybody who actually makes his or her own crackers. Only me. Menopause makes me do peculiar things. Cracker making is one of them. I can get one portion of plant estrogen from just one or two crackers. When I'm sick of flax bars and nutty snacks, I resort to whipping up a batch of crackers. Then I scoop up estrogenic dip or pâté on my little estrogenic concoctions.

FLAX CRACKERS

≋

Work and Cooking Time: *under 10 minutes*
Baking Time: *25 minutes*
Equipment: *electric coffee grinder*
Yield: *Makes 10 crackers*

Whisk ground flaxseed into warm soy milk and it instantly goes elastic. It can be stretched and rolled. It suddenly has the basic texture of pie dough. But it doesn't bake like pie dough. It stays elastic until it turns crisp—perfect for cracker making.

⅔ cup unsweetened soy milk
½ cup plus 2 tablespoons flaxseed
1 tablespoon brown miso

¼ cup whole-wheat flour, plus additional flour
for rolling

1. Preheat the oven to 325°F.
2. Bring the soy milk to a boil in a small saucepan. Remove from the heat.

3. Grind ½ cup of the flaxseed in an electric coffee grinder. Whisk into the hot soy milk. Stir in the miso and the 2 tablespoons of whole flaxseed. Add ¼ cup of whole-wheat flour to make a soft dough.

4. Sprinkle whole-wheat flour generously on a bread board. Turn the dough onto the floured board. Dust the dough generously with flour. Roll with a rolling pin to an 11×15-inch rectangle. If the dough becomes sticky, dust the board and dough with more flour.

5. Fold the dough and transfer it to an 11×15-inch nonstick or oiled cookie sheet. Unfold. Cut it into ten 5½×3-inch crackers: Cut the rolled dough in half lengthwise, then make five cuts 3 inches apart along the width of the pan. Bake for 25 minutes, until lightly browned and crisp.

PLANT ESTROGEN ESTIMATE: 1 PORTION PER CRACKER

RYE-CARAWAY CRACKERS

Work and Cooking Time: *under 10 minutes*
Baking Time: *30 minutes*
Equipment: *electric coffee grinder*
Yield: *Makes 10 crackers*

A very Scandinavian cracker.

⅔ cup unsweetened soy milk
½ cup flaxseed
1 tablespoon brown miso
2 tablespoons caraway seeds

¼ cup rye flour, plus additional flour for rolling

1. Preheat the oven to 325°F.
2. Bring the soy milk to a boil in a small saucepan. Remove from the heat.
3. Grind the flaxseed in an electric coffee grinder. Whisk into the hot soy milk. Stir in the miso and caraway seeds. Add ¼ cup of rye flour to make a soft dough.

4. Sprinkle rye flour generously on a bread board. Turn the dough onto the floured board. Dust the dough generously with flour. Roll with a rolling pin to an 11×15-inch rectangle. If the dough becomes sticky, dust the board and dough with more flour.

5. Fold the dough and transfer it to an 11×15-inch nonstick or oiled cookie sheet. Unfold. Cut it into twelve 5½×2½-inch crackers: Cut the rolled dough in half lengthwise, then make five cuts 2½ inches apart along the width of the pan. Bake for 30 minutes, until lightly browned and crisp.

> PLANT ESTROGEN ESTIMATE: ⅘ PORTION PER CRACKER

CORN CRACKERS

Work and Cooking Time: *under 10 minutes*
Baking Time: *25 minutes*
Equipment: *electric coffee grinder*
Yield: *Makes 32 crackers*

Darker and heavier than corn chips, these still make great guacamole or salsa dippers.

1⅓ cups unsweetened soy milk
1 cup flaxseed
1 tablespoon yellow miso

½ cup cornmeal, plus additional cornmeal for rolling

1. Preheat the oven to 325°F.

2. Bring the soy milk to a boil in a small saucepan. Remove from the heat.

3. Grind the flaxseed in an electric coffee grinder. Whisk into the hot soy milk. Stir in the miso and ½ cup of cornmeal to make a soft dough.

4. Divide the dough into four sections. Form into balls. Sprinkle cornmeal generously on a bread board. Turn the dough onto the floured board. Dust the dough generously with cornmeal. Roll with a rolling pin into four 8-inch circles.

5. Fold and transfer to four 8-inch nonstick or oiled cake pans. Cut each circle of dough into eight pizzalike pieces. Bake for 25 minutes, until lightly browned and crisp.

> PLANT ESTROGEN ESTIMATE: ½ PORTION PER CRACKER

TORTILLA BOWL

Work and Cooking Time: *under 10 minutes*
Baking Time: *30 minutes*
Equipment: *electric coffee grinder*
Yield: *Makes 1 serving*

Toss some salad in this tortilla bowl. Eat the salad. Then, eat the bowl!

½ cup unsweetened soy milk
⅓ cup flaxseed
2 teaspoons yellow miso

¼ cup cornmeal, plus additional cornmeal for rolling

1. Preheat the oven to 325°F.
2. Bring the soy milk to a boil in a small saucepan. Remove from the heat.
3. Grind the flaxseed in an electric coffee grinder. Whisk into the hot soy milk. Stir in the miso and ¼ cup of cornmeal to make a soft dough.
4. Form into a ball. Sprinkle cornmeal generously on a bread board. Turn the dough onto the floured board. Dust the dough generously with cornmeal. Roll with a rolling pin into a circle 15 inches in diameter.
5. Fold and transfer to an 11-inch nonstick or oiled pie plate. Unfold. Bake for 30 minutes, until lightly browned and crisp. Use as an edible container for salad.

PLANT ESTROGEN ESTIMATE: **6 PORTIONS PER SERVING**

≋ MUFFINS AND QUICK BREADS

Muffins without eggs, oil, or sugar—that's what you'll find in this section.

Sara, my younger daughter, mastered muffin making first—all my muffins turned to mush until she made the first deliciously moist batch. Flaxseed does a great job of replacing eggs and oil. Flaxseed infuses moisture—so much moisture that too much flaxseed creates permanent goo. To avoid overmoisturization when making flaxseed muffins and quick breads, you need to use enough flour and avoid underbaking. When the proportions and the cooking time are right, flaxseed-packed baked goods come out light and moist. No one would ever guess that you left out the oil and the eggs.

To replace the empty calories of sugar, these recipes rely on all-fruit jams and frozen juice concentrates. Both compress fruit, giving you a boost of the estrogenically friendly mineral boron.

For estrogenic baking, I try to pack as much flaxseed as possible into every muffin or slice. If you feel less compelled to maximize the amount of flaxseed, you can simply substitute eggs. One egg equals 1 tablespoon of ground flaxseed whisked into 3 tablespoons of water until it becomes slimy.

ORANGE-POPPY SEED MUFFINS

Work Time: *under 10 minutes*
Baking Time: *50 minutes*
Equipment: *electric blender*
Yield: *Makes 8 large muffins*

These muffins have the look of heavy health-food specimens. Bite into them, however, and you'll be surprised by their light, moist feel and their orange–poppy seed taste.

1¼ cups unbleached white flour

3 tablespoons soy flour

¼ cup poppy seeds

1 tablespoon baking soda

1 tablespoon grated orange rind

1½ cups soy milk

½ cup frozen orange juice concentrate

¼ cup all-fruit orange marmalade

⅓ cup flaxseed

1. Preheat the oven to 325°F.

2. Place all of the dry ingredients, including the orange rind, in a medium-size mixing bowl. Stir with a wire whisk until completely combined.

3. Place the soy milk, orange juice concentrate, orange marmalade, and flaxseed in an electric blender. Blend until the flaxseeds begin to disintegrate and the mixture bubbles. Pour into the dry ingredients. Stir to form a batter.

4. Spoon into eight nonstick or oiled large muffin tins. Bake for 50 minutes, until lightly browned.

PLANT ESTROGEN ESTIMATE: ⅞ PORTION PER MUFFIN

ALMOND-APRICOT MUFFINS

Work Time: *under 10 minutes*
Baking Time: *40 minutes*
Equipment: *electric blender*
Yield: *Makes 12 muffins*

Light, moist, and sweet—without eggs, oil, or sugar!

2 cups unbleached white flour	2 cups soy milk
⅓ cup soy flour	½ cup frozen orange juice concentrate
2 teaspoons grated orange rind	2 tablespoons almond extract
2 teaspoons baking soda	½ cup all-fruit apricot jam
1 cup chopped dried apricots	½ cup flaxseed

1. Preheat the oven to 325°F.

2. Place all of the dry ingredients, including the orange rind, in a medium-size mixing bowl. Stir with a wire whisk until completely combined. Add the apricots. Stir in.

3. Place the remaining ingredients in an electric blender. Blend until the flaxseeds begin to disintegrate and the mixture bubbles. Pour into the dry ingredients. Stir to form a batter.

4. Spoon into twelve nonstick or oiled muffin tins, filling to the top. Bake for 40 minutes, until browned and firm to the touch.

PLANT ESTROGEN ESTIMATE: 1 PORTION PER MUFFIN

APPLE-RAISIN-SPICE MUFFINS

Work Time: *under 10 minutes*
Baking Time: *40 minutes*
Equipment: *electric blender*
Yield: *Makes 12 muffins*

Like carrot muffins, without the carrots.

2 cups unbleached white flour
⅓ cup soy flour
3 tablespoons ground cinnamon
1 teaspoon ground nutmeg
2 teaspoons grated orange rind
2 teaspoons baking soda
1 cup chopped dried apples

1 cup raisins
2 cups soy milk
½ cup frozen orange juice concentrate
½ cup all-fruit orange marmalade
½ cup flaxseed

1. Preheat the oven to 325°F.

2. Place all of the dry ingredients, including the orange rind, in a medium-size mixing bowl. Stir with a wire whisk until completely combined. Add the apple and raisins. Stir in.

3. Place the remaining ingredients in an electric blender. Blend until the flaxseeds begin to disintegrate and the mixture bubbles. Pour into the dry ingredients. Stir to form a batter.

4. Spoon into twelve nonstick or oiled muffin tins, filling to the top. Bake for 40 minutes, until browned and firm to the touch.

PLANT ESTROGEN ESTIMATE: 1 PORTION PER MUFFIN

BANANA-NUT MINI-MUFFINS

Work Time: *under 10 minutes*
Baking Time: *40 minutes*
Equipment: *electric blender*
Yield: *Makes 24 mini-muffins*

Thanks go to natural banana flavor for the taste of these not-too-sweet muffins. One banana gives only a hint of banana taste. More than one banana makes for pastelike insides. Natural banana flavor is the perfect solution.

2 cups unbleached white flour
⅓ cup soy flour
2 teaspoons baking soda
2 cups soy milk
1 banana, sliced
½ cup all-fruit apricot jam

1 tablespoon vanilla extract
3 tablespoons natural banana flavor
2 tablespoons lemon juice
½ cup flaxseed
⅔ cup coarsely chopped walnuts

1. Preheat the oven to 325°F.

2. Place all of the dry ingredients in a medium-size mixing bowl. Stir with a wire whisk until completely combined.

3. Place the remaining ingredients, except the walnuts, in an electric blender. Blend until the flaxseeds begin to disintegrate and the mixture bubbles. Pour into the dry ingredients. Stir to form a batter. Add the walnuts and stir to combine.

4. Spoon into twenty-four nonstick or oiled mini-muffin tins, filling to the top. Bake for 40 minutes, until browned and firm to the touch.

PLANT ESTROGEN ESTIMATE: NEARLY ½ PORTION PER MUFFIN

NINA SHANDLER

DATE-NUT BREAD

Work Time: *under 10 minutes*
Baking Time: *1 ½ hours*
Equipment: *electric coffee grinder*
Yield: *Makes 12 servings*

Just your basic high-protein, estrogen-rich date-nut loaf.

½ cup flaxseed

2¼ cups soy milk

1 tablespoon vanilla extract

3 cups whole-wheat pastry flour

⅔ cup soy flour

½ cup raw sugar

2 tablespoons baking powder

1 tablespoon ground cinnamon

1 cup chopped dates

⅔ cup coarsely chopped walnuts

1. Preheat the oven to 300°F.

2. Grind the flaxseed in an electric coffee grinder. Place in a bowl. Add the soy milk and vanilla. Whisk together. Set aside.

3. Place the pastry flour, soy flour, sugar, baking powder, and cinnamon in a mixing bowl. Stir with a wire whisk until well combined. Add the flax–and–soy milk mixture. Stir to form a batter. Fold in the dates and nuts. Turn into a 9×5-inch nonstick or oiled loaf pan.

4. Bake for 1½ hours, until lightly browned. Remove from the pan to cool.

PLANT ESTROGEN ESTIMATE: 1 PORTION PER SERVING

CORN BREAD

Work Time: *under 10 minutes*
Baking Time: *1 hour*
Equipment: *electric coffee grinder*
Yield: *Makes 9 servings*

This bread goes well with chili, pea soup, or gumbo.

½ cup flaxseed

1½ cups soy milk

½ cup frozen apple juice concentrate

1¼ cups cornmeal

⅓ cup soy flour

1½ tablespoons baking powder

¼ teaspoon salt

1. Preheat the oven to 300°F.

2. Grind the flaxseed in an electric coffee grinder. Place in a bowl. Add the soy milk and apple juice concentrate. Whisk together. Set aside.

3. Place the remaining ingredients in a mixing bowl. Stir with a wire whisk until well combined. Add the flax–and–soy milk mixture. Stir to form a batter. Turn into a 9×9-inch nonstick or oiled pan.

4. Bake for 1 hour, until lightly browned. Remove from the pan to cool. Cut into nine squares to serve.

PLANT ESTROGEN ESTIMATE: 1 PORTION PER SERVING

BROWN BREAD

Work Time: *under 10 minutes*
Baking Time: *1½ hours*
Equipment: *electric coffee grinder*
Yield: *Makes 12 servings*

Inspired by a sweet tradition—brown bread with Boston baked beans—this loaf is a lighter brown than the original. Feel free to break with tradition. It makes great raisin toast.

½ cup flaxseed	⅔ cup soy flour
2½ cups soy milk	2 tablespoons baking powder
⅓ cup blackstrap molasses	½ teaspoon salt
3 cups whole-wheat pastry flour	1 cup raisins

1. Preheat the oven to 300°F.

2. Grind the flaxseed in an electric coffee grinder. Place in a bowl. Add the soy milk and molasses. Whisk together. Set aside.

3. Place the pastry flour, soy flour, baking powder, and salt in a mixing bowl. Stir with a wire whisk until well combined. Add the flax–and–soy milk mixture. Stir to form a batter. Fold in the raisins. Turn into a 9×5-inch nonstick or oiled loaf pan.

4. Bake for 1½ hours, until lightly browned. Remove from the pan to cool.

> **PLANT ESTROGEN ESTIMATE: 1 PORTION PER SERVING**

YEAST BREADS

Some people need to knead. You're groaning. I know you're groaning, but I just couldn't resist saying it. Anyway, if you love bread making, here are a few estrogenically enriched recipes. The big challenge is to figure out how much flaxseed you can cram into a recipe without creating a concoction that resembles moist rubber. My basic proportion for yeast bread is at least two and a half times as much flour as flax. There's a great payoff from getting the proportions right: Flaxseed bread doesn't dry out. It tastes and feels fresh days longer than other breads.

CARAWAY-RYE BREAD

Work Time: *under 30 minutes*
Rising Time: *1½ hours*
Baking Time: *1½ hours*
Equipment: *electric blender*
Yield: *Makes 2 loaves of 10 slices each*

Tastes like a classic.

½ cup lukewarm soy milk
1 tablespoon maple syrup
1 tablespoon granulated yeast
1¾ cups flaxseed
¼ cup dark miso
2½ cups soy milk, at room temperature, plus additional milk for coating the loaves

¼ cup caraway seeds
1 cup soy flour
1 cup unbleached white flour
1 cup rye flour
1½ cups whole-wheat flour
Canola-oil spray

1. In a large stoneware bowl, combine the lukewarm soy milk and maple syrup. Sprinkle the yeast over the mixture.

2. In an electric blender, blend the flaxseed, miso, and the 2½ cups soy milk for 4 minutes, until the mixture thickens and bubbles. Pour into the bowl with the dissolved yeast. Beat together with a wooden spoon. Beat in the caraway seeds, soy flour, and white flour one ingredient at a time. Cover the bowl. Place in a warm spot to rise for about 45 minutes, until doubled in bulk.

3. Using a wooden spoon, stir in the rye flour. Measure ½ cup whole-wheat flour onto a bread board. Turn the dough onto the board and knead in the remaining whole-wheat flour ½ cup at a time. Form into two oval-shaped loaves. Place them on a nonstick or

oiled cookie sheet. Cover and allow to rise in a warm place for another 45 minutes, until doubled in bulk.

4. Preheat the oven to 325°F. Using a pastry brush, coat the loaves with soy milk. Bake for 1½ hours, until the crust is brown. Spray with oil. Allow to cool on a rack.

PLANT ESTROGEN ESTIMATE: 1¾ PORTIONS PER SLICE

WHOLE-WHEAT BREAD

Work Time: *under 30 minutes*
Rising Time: *1½ hours*
Baking Time: *1½ hours*
Equipment: *electric coffee grinder*
Yield: *Makes 2 loaves of 10 slices each*

I hear they use lots of flaxseed in Africa. I believe it's a basic ingredient in African bread.

Michael, my husband, grew up in South Africa. He ate the same bread every day for the first nineteen years of his life. He left. He craved the bread. Over and over, at bakery after bakery, in country after country, he bought cracked-wheat bread. But no bread measured up. Then, in a morning of estrogen-seeking activity, I made this flaxseed bread. It was *the bread.* He consumed the whole loaf in one sitting.

½ cup lukewarm soy milk
1 tablespoon raw sugar
1 tablespoon granulated yeast
1¾ cups flaxseed
2½ cups soy milk, at room temperature, plus
   additional milk for coating the loaves

¼ cup dark miso
1 cup soy flour
3½ cups whole-wheat flour

1. In a small bowl, combine the lukewarm soy milk and sugar. Sprinkle the yeast over the mixture.

2. Grind the flaxseed in an electric coffee grinder ⅓ cup at a time. Pour it into a large stoneware bowl. Using a wire whisk, beat in the 2½ cups of soy milk and the miso. Add

the dissolved-yeast mixture. Whisk until the miso is fully dissolved and the mixture has thickened. Stir in the soy flour. Beat in 1 cup of whole-wheat flour. Cover the bowl. Place in a warm spot to rise for about 45 minutes, until doubled in bulk.

3. Using a wooden spoon, stir in ½ cup of whole-wheat flour. Measure ½ cup of whole-wheat flour onto a bread board. Turn the dough onto the board and knead in the remaining whole-wheat flour ½ cup at a time until the dough is no longer sticky. Form into two oval-shaped loaves. Place them on a nonstick or oiled cookie sheet. Cover and allow to rise in a warm place for another 45 minutes, until doubled in bulk.

4. Preheat the oven to 325°F. Using a pastry brush, coat the loaves with soy milk. Bake for 1½ hours, until the crust is brown. Allow to cool on a rack.

PLANT ESTROGEN ESTIMATE: 1¾ PORTIONS PER SLICE

CARDAMOM ROLLS

Work Time: *under 40 minutes*
Rising Time: *1½ hours*
Baking Time: *1¼ hours*
Equipment: *electric coffee grinder*
Yield: *Makes 9 servings*

A special bread for special occasions, these sweet cardamom rolls dress up any dinner party.

½ cup lukewarm soy milk
½ cup maple syrup
1 tablespoon granulated yeast
1 cup flaxseed
1¾ cups soy milk, at room temperature, plus
    additional milk for coating the rolls

3 tablespoons yellow miso
3 tablespoons ground cardamom
¾ cup soy flour
3¾ cups unbleached white flour
Raw sugar
Canola-oil spray

1. In a small bowl, combine the lukewarm soy milk and maple syrup. Sprinkle the yeast over the mixture.

2. Grind the flaxseed in an electric coffee grinder ⅓ cup at a time. Pour it into a large stoneware bowl. Using a wire whisk, beat in the 1¾ cups of soy milk, the miso, and the cardamom. Add the dissolved-yeast mixture. Whisk until the miso is fully dissolved and the mixture has thickened. Stir in the soy flour. Beat in 1¼ cups of white flour. Cover the bowl. Place in a warm spot to rise for about 45 minutes, until doubled in bulk.

3. Using a wooden spoon, stir in 1 cup of white flour. Measure ½ cup of flour onto a bread board. Turn the dough onto the board and knead in the remaining flour ½ cup at a time until the dough is no longer sticky.

4. Form into nine balls. Place them evenly spaced in a 9×9-inch nonstick or oiled cake pan. Cover and allow to rise in a warm place for another 45 minutes, until doubled in bulk.

5. Preheat the oven to 325°F. Using a pastry brush, coat the rolls with soy milk. Bake for 1 to 1¼ hours, until the crust is brown. Remove from the oven. Sprinkle with raw sugar. Spray with oil. Remove from the pan and cool on a rack.

PLANT ESTROGEN ESTIMATE: 2⅓ PORTIONS PER SERVING

CINNAMON-RAISIN BREAD

Working Time: *under 30 minutes*
Rising Time: *1½ hours*
Baking Time: *1½ hours*
Equipment: *electric coffee grinder*
Yield: *Makes 2 loaves of 10 slices per loaf*

Subtly sweet—the perfect morning toast.

½ cup table molasses
1 tablespoon blackstrap molasses
3 cups lukewarm soy milk, plus additional
   milk for coating the loaves
1 tablespoon granulated yeast
3 tablespoons yellow miso

1¾ cups flaxseed
¼ cup ground cinnamon
1 cup raisins
1 cup soy flour
3 to 3½ cups whole-wheat flour

1. In a large stoneware bowl, combine the table molasses, blackstrap molasses, and lukewarm soy milk. Sprinkle the yeast over the mixture. Allow to sit for 5 minutes, until yeast has dissolved. Whisk in the miso, making sure it dissolves completely.

2. Grind the flaxseed in an electric coffee grinder ⅓ cup at a time. Add to the yeast–and–soy milk mixture. Using a wire whisk, beat until the mixture thickens. Whisk in the cinnamon. Using a wooden spoon, stir in the raisins. Stir in the soy flour and 1 cup of whole-wheat flour. Mix until well combined. Cover the bowl. Place in a warm spot to rise for about 45 minutes, until doubled in bulk.

3. Using a wooden spoon, stir in ½ cup of whole-wheat flour. Measure ½ cup of whole-wheat flour onto a bread board. Turn the dough onto the board and knead in the remaining whole-wheat flour ½ cup at a time until the dough is no longer sticky.

4. Form into two oval-shaped loaves. Place them on a nonstick or oiled cookie sheet. Cover and allow to rise in a warm place for another 45 minutes, until doubled in bulk.

5. Preheat the oven to 325°F. Using a pastry brush, coat the loaves with soy milk. Bake for 1½ hours, until the crust is brown. Allow to cool on a rack.

PLANT ESTROGEN ESTIMATE: 1¾ PORTIONS PER SLICE

PECAN STICKY BUNS

Work Time: *under 40 minutes*
Rising Time: *1½ hours*
Baking Time: *45 minutes*
Equipment: *electric blender and electric coffee grinder*
Yield: *Makes 6 rolls*

These are very sticky but not too sweet. Serve them for breakfast, dinner, or in between.

½ cup lukewarm soy milk

½ cup maple syrup

1 tablespoon granulated yeast

1½ cups soy milk, at room temperature, plus additional milk for coating the buns

2 tablespoons yellow miso

1 cup flaxseed

¾ cup soy flour

¼ cup plus 2 teaspoons ground cinnamon

3¼ cups unbleached white flour

⅓ cup brown-rice syrup

⅓ cup barley malt

¾ cup coarsely chopped pecans

Canola-oil spray

1. In a small bowl, combine the lukewarm soy milk and maple syrup. Sprinkle the yeast over the mixture.

2. Pour the 1½ cups of soy milk into an electric blender. Add the miso. Grind the flaxseed in an electric coffee grinder ⅓ cup at a time and add to the ingredients in the blender. Blend at high speed until the mixture thickens and bubbles. Pour into a large stoneware bowl. Stir in the dissolved-yeast mixture. Using a wooden spoon, beat in the soy flour, ¼ cup of cinnamon, and 1 cup of the unbleached white flour. Cover the bowl. Place in a warm spot to rise for about 45 minutes, until doubled in bulk.

3. Using a wooden spoon, stir in 1 cup of white flour. Measure ½ cup of flour onto a bread board. Turn the dough onto the board and knead in the remaining flour ½ cup at a time until the dough is no longer sticky. Flour the board. Using a floured rolling pin, roll the dough into a 10×12-inch rectangle.

4. Heat the rice syrup and malt in a small, heavy-bottomed saucepan just until liquid. Spread the warm syrup over the dough. Sprinkle with the 2 teaspoons of cinnamon and the pecans. Cut the dough into six 10×2-inch strips. Roll the strips loosely. Pinch one end of each strip. Place them in popover-size nonstick or oiled muffin tins with the pinched ends down. Place in a warm spot. Cover and allow to rise for 45 minutes, until doubled in bulk.

5. Preheat the oven to 325°F. Using a pastry brush, coat the tops of the buns with soy milk. Bake for 45 minutes, until the crust is brown. Spray with oil. Remove from the tins and cool on a rack.

PLANT ESTROGEN ESTIMATE: 3 PORTIONS PER ROLL

Six

Soups

Maybe it's because I grew up on Campbell's soup ads. When I start thinking about soup, only really corny sentiments come to mind—like "soup soothes the soul." Or "from creamy cold to steamy hot, from summer to winter, soups give warmth and nourishment." At any rate, soup really works well for a lunch, a light dinner, or an appetizer. All of these soups come with a fringe benefit—extra estrogen.

≋ CHILLED SOUPS

When the days turn humid or the hot flashes turn intrusive, sip cold soup to ease the heat. I love to serve these soups on a summer day, outside, with the flowers blooming. For chilled creamy soups, keep your blender handy, ready to whip up a refreshing lunch, a light dinner, or an appealing appetizer.

CHILLED TOMATO BISQUE

Work Time: *under 5 minutes*
Equipment: *electric blender*
Yield: *Makes 4 servings*

A creamy cold tomato bisque. For a more elegant soup, add some cold shrimp or scallops.

4 garlic cloves, pressed

1 cup soy milk

1 cake (19 ounces) silken tofu

3 tablespoons finely chopped fresh basil or
   cilantro

⅛ teaspoon salt

¾ cup tomato sauce

Fresh herb garnish

Place all of the ingredients in an electric blender and blend until smooth. Taste. If needed, add more salt, basil, or cilantro. Pour into four soup bowls and garnish with fresh herbs. Serve.

PLANT ESTROGEN ESTIMATE: 1¼ PORTIONS PER SERVING

VICHYSSOISE

Work and Cooking Time: *15 minutes*
Equipment: *electric food processor*
Yield: *Makes 4 servings*

Every bit as creamy as traditional vichyssoise, this is protein-packed, estrogen-rich, and low in fat.

3 new potatoes, diced

1 onion

2 bay leaves

3 tablespoons chopped fresh parsley

⅓ cup chopped scallion

½ cake (9½ ounces) silken tofu

2 cups soy milk

Salt and pepper

1. Steam the potatoes, onion, and bay leaves until the potatoes are soft.

2. Remove the bay leaves and place the potatoes and onion in a food processor with the S blade inserted. Add the parsley, scallion, and tofu. Process until smooth.

3. Pour the purée into a serving bowl. Whisk in the soy milk. Season with salt and pepper. Serve.

PLANT ESTROGEN ESTIMATE: 1 PORTION PER SERVING

COLD CREAMY CUCUMBER SOUP

Work Time: *under 10 minutes*
Equipment: *electric food processor*
Yield: *Makes 4 servings*

This soup is my favorite summer lunch.

6 garlic cloves, quartered
⅔ cup sliced scallion
1 cup fresh cilantro leaves
½ cup fresh mint leaves
1 cake (19 ounces) silken tofu

⅓ cup yellow miso
¼ cup lemon juice
3 cups soy milk
1 English cucumber, grated

1. Place the garlic in a food processor with the S blade inserted. Add the scallion, cilantro, and mint. Mince. Add the tofu, miso, and lemon juice. Process until smooth. Taste. If needed, add more cilantro or mint.

2. Pour into a serving bowl. Whisk in the soy milk. Stir in the cucumber. Serve.

PLANT ESTROGEN ESTIMATE: 1¾ PORTIONS PER SERVING

AVOCADO SOUP

Work Time: *under 10 minutes*
Equipment: *electric food processor*
Yield: *Makes 4 servings*

Avocado and tofu combine for a smooth, rich texture. Be sure to use *unsweetened* soy milk; sweetened soy milk would add an odd note to this refreshing soup.

6 garlic cloves, quartered

½ cup sliced scallion

½ cup fresh cilantro leaves

⅓ cup lemon juice

2 avocados, peeled and sliced

1 cake (19 ounces) silken tofu

3 cups unsweetened soy milk

Salt

¼ cup salsa

1. Place the garlic in a food processor with the S blade inserted. Mince. Add the scallion and cilantro. Mince. Add the lemon juice, avocados, and tofu. Process until smooth and creamy.

2. Pour into a large mixing bowl. Whisk in the soy milk. Salt to taste. If needed, add more lemon. Ladle into four soup bowls. Place 1 tablespoon of salsa in the center of each serving.

PLANT ESTROGEN ESTIMATE: 1¾ PORTIONS PER SERVING

CURRIED APPLE SOUP

Work Time: *under 10 minutes*
Equipment: *electric food processor*
Yield: *Makes 4 servings*

I served this sweet and spicy apple soup on my fiftieth birthday. It was a hit!

3 garlic cloves, quartered

2 tablespoons curry powder

1½ teaspoons ground cinnamon

¼ teaspoon turmeric

½ cup frozen apple juice concentrate

1 cake (19 ounces) silken tofu

3 cups soy milk

4 apples, grated

⅓ cup raisins

1. Place the garlic in a food processor with the S blade inserted. Mince. Add the curry powder, cinnamon, turmeric, apple juice concentrate, and tofu. Process until smooth and creamy.

2. Pour into a serving bowl. Whisk in the soy milk. Stir in the grated apple and raisins. Taste. If needed, add more curry powder. Serve.

PLANT ESTROGEN ESTIMATE: 1¾ PORTIONS PER SERVING

CREAMY COLD STRAWBERRY SOUP

Work Time: *under 10 minutes*
Equipment: *electric blender*
Yield: *Makes 4 servings*

Another of Sara's favorites. When a teenager says, "Mom, you can make this anytime," it must be good.

2 cups strawberries, fresh or frozen

2 tablespoons vanilla extract

2 tablespoons all-fruit strawberry jam

½ cup frozen apple juice concentrate

1 cake (19 ounces) silken tofu

2 cups soy milk

Place all of the ingredients in an electric blender. Blend until smooth. Taste. If needed, add more vanilla. Serve.

PLANT ESTROGEN ESTIMATE: 1¾ PORTIONS PER SERVING

BLUEBERRY SOUP WITH STRAWBERRIES

Work Time: *under 10 minutes*
Equipment: *electric blender*
Yield: *Makes 4 servings*

Want a fabulous-looking soup? Choose this one—it's electric purple with a red-pink strawberry center.

3 cups frozen blueberries
1 cup frozen white grape juice concentrate
1 cake (19 ounces) silken tofu

1 cup soy milk
1 teaspoon ground nutmeg
1 cup sliced fresh strawberries

Place the frozen blueberries, grape juice concentrate, tofu, soy milk, and nutmeg in an electric blender. Blend until smooth. Taste. If needed, add more nutmeg. Pour into a serving bowl. Spoon the strawberries into the middle. Serve.

> **PLANT ESTROGEN ESTIMATE: 1¼ PORTIONS PER SERVING**

HOT AND HEARTY SOUPS

When my children get sick or when my husband's in bed, the soup goes on the burner. At our house, we believe in the healing power of hot soup. In this section you'll find flavorful medicine to protect you from cold-weather ills—all estrogen-inoculated.

CURRIED PUMPKIN BISQUE

Work and Cooking Time: *under 15 minutes*
Equipment: *electric food processor*
Yield: *Makes 6 servings*

15-ounce can solid-pack pumpkin

2 cups soy milk

3 garlic cloves, quartered

4 ⅛×1-inch slices fresh ginger

1 cake (19 ounces) silken tofu

¼ cup frozen apple juice concentrate

2 teaspoons curry powder

Salt

1 tablespoon chopped fresh cilantro

1. Whisk the pumpkin and soy milk together in a soup pot. Cook over medium heat.

2. Place the garlic in a food processor with the S blade inserted. Mince. Add the ginger. Mince. Add the tofu. Process until smooth.

3. Add the tofu mixture to the soup pot. Whisk until blended. Stir in the apple juice concentrate and curry powder. Cook until hot, without boiling. Salt to taste.

4. Ladle into soup bowls and garnish with cilantro.

PLANT ESTROGEN ESTIMATE: 1 PORTION PER SERVING

NEW ENGLAND FISH CHOWDER

Work and Cooking Time: *20 minutes*
Equipment: *electric food processor*
Yield: *Makes 4 servings*

This tastes like a prize-winning heavy-cream concoction. No one will ever know you left out the cream, the cholesterol, and the excess calories. By the way, cod, like tofu, is a great calcium source.

Take care not to boil this chowder. Even a little bubble will cause it to curdle. The texture will change from creamy to coagulated. It will still be okay, but it will be far from great.

2 potatoes, peeled and diced	½ cup soy milk
1 onion, chopped	8 ounces cod
3 garlic cloves, pressed	Salt and pepper
1 teaspoon dill seeds	Pinch fresh dill
1 cake (19 ounces) silken tofu	

1. Place the potatoes and 1 cup of water in a soup pot. Bring to a boil. When the potatoes can be pierced easily with a fork, reduce the heat to medium. Add the onion, garlic, and dill seeds.

2. Purée the tofu and soy milk in a food processor with the S blade inserted. Pour into the soup pot and cook over medium-low heat without bringing to a boil. Cut the fish into 1-inch chunks. Add to the soup pot. Continue cooking without boiling until the fish is fully cooked. Add salt and pepper to taste.

3. Garnish with a pinch of dill before serving.

PLANT ESTROGEN ESTIMATE: 1⅛ PORTIONS PER SERVING

GREEK-STYLE LEMON SOUP

Work and Cooking Time: *under 20 minutes*
Equipment: *electric blender*
Yield: *Makes 4 servings*

Cooked to perfection, this soup has a lightly creamy texture. If it's left on the burner too long, it thickens and becomes gravy. To correct, just stir in water.

Stir the lemon into the soup just before serving. Otherwise, it's very likely to curdle. If you want leftovers, refrigerate the soup without adding the lemon; add it after you reheat the creamy base.

½ cup orzo

3½ cups unsweetened soy milk

¼ cake (4½ ounces) silken tofu

8 garlic cloves, pressed

⅔ cup lemon juice

Salt

2 tablespoons chopped fresh cilantro

1. Measure the orzo into 2 quarts of boiling water. Cook for 10 minutes.

2. While the orzo is cooking, prepare the broth: Place the soy milk and tofu in an electric blender. Blend until smooth. Add the garlic. Blend to mix thoroughly.

3. Pour the creamy broth into a heavy-bottomed soup pot. Cook over medium heat. When the orzo is fully cooked, drain and add to the cooking soup broth.

4. Remove from the heat and stir in the lemon juice. Salt to taste. If needed, add more lemon and salt. Ladle into soup bowls and sprinkle with chopped cilantro.

PLANT ESTROGEN ESTIMATE: 1 PORTION PER SERVING

CAJUN-STYLE GUMBO

Work and Cooking Time: *under 20 minutes*

Yield: *Makes 6 servings*

Just a little soy flour thickens this classic Cajun soup without changing its tomato-red color. Whole flaxseed works in this recipe. It mimics the slightly slimy texture of okra. Soy sausage delivers a full-bodied taste and a full measure of plant estrogens. And miso makes the broth more meatlike.

Spray oil

3 garlic cloves, minced

1 medium onion, chopped

10 soy sausages, sliced

10-ounce package frozen okra, thawed and
    rinsed

½ green bell pepper, diced

28-ounce can diced tomatoes

1 teaspoon dried thyme

2 tablespoons dark miso

1 tablespoon flaxseed

⅓ cup soy flour

1. Spray a heavy-bottomed soup pot lightly with oil. (If available, mesquite-flavored olive oil tastes great in this dish.) Heat the soup pot over medium-high heat. Sauté the garlic, onion, and sausage. When the onion is browned, add the okra, green bell pepper, tomatoes, thyme, miso, and flaxseed.

2. Dissolve the soy flour in 2 cups of water. Add to the soup pot. Cook until the soup is hot and the broth has thickened slightly. Serve.

PLANT ESTROGEN ESTIMATE: 1 PORTION PER SERVING

BORSCHT

Work and Cooking Time: *20 minutes*
Equipment: *electric food processor*
Yield: *Makes 4 servings*

A traditional beet borscht with a twist of ginger. Go heavy on the creamy ginger topping—it has most of the plant estrogens.

Soup	Topping
4 new potatoes	½-inch slice fresh ginger
4 beets, grated	1 garlic clove, quartered
3 tablespoons yellow miso	½ cake (8 ounces) soft tofu
1 teaspoon apple cider vinegar	Salt

1. Place the potatoes in a soup pot with 3 cups of water. Bring to a boil. When the potatoes can be pierced with a fork, reduce the heat to medium. Add the grated beets, miso, and vinegar.

2. While the borscht cooks, make the topping: Chop the ginger into ¼-inch chunks. Place in a food processor with the S blade inserted. Mince. Add the garlic. Mince. Add the tofu. Process for 3 minutes, until the tofu is smooth, with no grainy texture. Salt to taste.

3. Remove the soup from the stove. Serve with the topping.

PLANT ESTROGEN ESTIMATE: ⅔ PORTION PER SERVING

ROASTED GARLIC, WHITE BEAN, AND SAUSAGE SOUP

Work and Cooking Time: *under 15 minutes*
Equipment: *electric food processor*
Yield: *Makes 4 servings*

Creamy without cream. Soy sausage, tofu, and soy milk provide natural estrogens. To save time, I use bottled roasted garlic cloves.

Spray oil
10 soy sausages, sliced
3 garlic cloves, quartered
1 cake (16 ounces) soft tofu
2 tablespoons whole roasted garlic cloves
2 tablespoons dark miso

15-ounce can white or great northern beans, drained
1½ cups unsweetened soy milk
¼ cup chopped roasted garlic cloves
1 tablespoon mustard seed
Pepper

1. Spray a heavy-bottomed soup pot with oil. Sauté the sliced sausage over medium-high heat.

2. While the sausage sautés, place the fresh garlic in a food processor with the S blade inserted. Mince. Add the tofu, 2 tablespoons roasted garlic, and miso. Process for 2 minutes, until smooth and silky.

3. Add the tofu mixture, the beans, soy milk, ¼ cup chopped roasted garlic, and mustard seed to the sausage. Reduce the heat to medium and stir until all of the ingredients are well combined. Cook, stirring occasionally, without bringing to a boil, until heated through. Season with pepper before serving.

PLANT ESTROGEN ESTIMATE: **2** PORTIONS PER SERVING

BASIC BISQUE

Work and Cooking Time: *15 minutes*
Equipment: *electric food processor*
Yield: *Makes 4 servings*

A pretty pink tomato soup with a touch of cinnamon may sound disgusting, but it's a favorite at our house. I learned to combine these flavors from Indian cooking. Sara, my younger daughter, approves. She says, "Tell them I like the creamy tomato soup a lot." She especially likes it with a little added indulgence: A few shrimps or scallops transform this simple soup into an elegant seafood bisque.

Remember—tofu will curdle just like milk. Stir the tofu purée in at the very end, being careful not to overheat. Also, if you substitute ground cinnamon for cinnamon sticks, the color will change from pretty pink to drab brown.

15-ounce can tomato sauce	1 cake (19 ounces) silken tofu
6 cinnamon sticks	½ cup soy milk
3 garlic cloves, quartered	Ground cinnamon
6 ⅛×1-inch slices fresh ginger	

1. Combine the tomato sauce and 1 cup of water in a soup pot. Add the cinnamon sticks. Cook over medium heat.

2. Place the garlic and ginger in a food processor with the S blade inserted. Mince. Add the minced garlic and ginger to the cooking tomato stock. Allow to simmer for 10 minutes.

3. While the tomato stock simmers, place the tofu and soy milk in the food processor. Process until smooth and silky.

4. Remove the tomato stock from the burner. Stir in the tofu mixture. Sprinkle with ground cinnamon and serve.

PLANT ESTROGEN ESTIMATE: 1¼ PORTIONS PER SERVING

MEXICAN-STYLE BLACK BEAN-AND-BACIN SOUP

Work and Cooking Time: *under 10 minutes*
Equipment: *electric food processor*
Yield: *Makes 4 servings*

In Puerto Vallarta, black bean soup is served with small side dishes of sour cream, chopped onion, minced jalapeño pepper, and sliced lime. Diners add as much or as little of each as suits their taste. This black bean soup parts with tradition. To increase natural estrogen and decrease mouth-burning heat, it's served with a lemon-garlic tofu topping, chopped onion, and minced fresh cilantro.

Soup
29-ounce can black beans
4 garlic cloves, pressed
2 tablespoons bacin bits
1 tablespoon dark miso

Garnish
4 tablespoons chopped fresh cilantro
1 small onion, chopped

Topping
2 garlic cloves, quartered
½ cake (8 ounces) soft tofu
2 tablespoons lemon juice
Salt

1. Combine the beans, 1 cup of water, garlic, bacin bits, and miso in a soup pot. Cook over medium-high heat.

2. While the beans are cooking, prepare the tofu topping: Place the garlic in a food processor with the S blade inserted. Mince. Add the tofu and lemon juice. Process for 2 minutes, until smooth and silky. Salt to taste. Place the tofu topping in a small serving dish.

3. Place the cilantro and onion in separate small serving dishes.

4. Ladle the soup into bowls. Serve with topping, onion, and cilantro.

PLANT ESTROGEN ESTIMATE: ¾ PORTION PER SERVING

PORTOBELLO MUSHROOM SOUP

Work and Cooking Time: *under 10 minutes*
Equipment: *electric food processor*
Yield: *Makes 6 servings*

Michael and I had our first creamy portobello mushroom soup in a very classy Italian restaurant and bar on the Upper West Side of Manhattan. When we got home we wanted more. I got to work in the kitchen. The result is this very satisfying estrogenic version with a rich, earthy portobello flavor and a creamy feel.

Spray oil
1 pound portobello mushrooms, chopped
3 garlic cloves, pressed
1 cake (19 ounces) silken tofu

½ teaspoon ground cumin
2 tablespoons dark miso
2 cups soy milk

1. Spray a frying pan with oil and sauté the mushrooms until browned.
2. Place the mushrooms, garlic, tofu, cumin, and miso in a food processor with the S blade inserted. Process until smooth.
3. Turn the mixture into a soup pot. Whisk in the soy milk. Taste. Add more cumin if needed. Heat over medium-high heat. When the soup simmers, remove it from the heat.

PLANT ESTROGEN ESTIMATE: 1 PORTION PER SERVING

SPINACH POTAGE

Work and Cooking Time: *under 15 minutes*
Equipment: *electric food processor*
Yield: *Makes 4 servings*

Spinach with a hint of ginger gives this bright-green French-style soup an Indian flavor.

Spray oil
1 large onion, chopped
4 garlic cloves, chopped
4 ⅛×1-inch slices fresh ginger
16 ounces fresh spinach, steamed, or frozen
 spinach, thawed

1 cake (19 ounces) silken tofu
1½ cups soy milk
3 tablespoons lemon juice
Salt

1. Spray a frying pan with oil. Sauté the onion, garlic, and ginger until browned. Place in a food processor with the S blade inserted. Add the spinach and tofu. Process until smooth.

2. Turn the mixture into a soup pot. Stir in the soy milk. Cook over medium-high heat.

3. When hot, remove from the heat and stir in the lemon juice. Salt to taste.

PLANT ESTROGEN ESTIMATE: 1¾ PORTIONS PER SERVING

GINGER-CARROT SOUP

Work and Cooking Time: *under 15 minutes*
Equipment: *electric food processor*
Yield: *Makes 4 servings*

Electric orange with a spicy sweetness, this soup is a carrot lover's delight.

8 carrots, sliced
7 ⅛×1-inch slices fresh ginger
4 garlic cloves

½ cake (8 ounces) soft tofu
3 tablespoons yellow miso
3 cups soy milk

1. Pour ½ cup of water into a soup pot. Add the carrots, ginger, and garlic. Cook over high heat until the carrots are soft.

2. Place the cooked carrot mixture in a food processor with the S blade inserted. Add the tofu and miso. Process until smooth. Return to the soup pot. Stir in the soy milk. Reduce the heat to medium. Cook until hot.

PLANT ESTROGEN ESTIMATE: 1⅓ PORTIONS PER SERVING

SWEET POTATO-DILL SOUP

Work and Cooking Time: *under 25 minutes*
Equipment: *electric food processor*
Yield: *Makes 4 servings*

Orange with flecks of green—a feast for the eyes as well as the palate.

1 large peeled sweet potato or yam, cut into
   1-inch chunks
4 garlic cloves, quartered
2 tablespoons yellow miso

½ cake (8 ounces) soft tofu
3 cups soy milk
2 tablespoons snipped fresh dill
2 tablespoons lemon juice

1. Pour ½ cup of water into a soup pot. Add the sweet potato and garlic. Cook over high heat until the sweet potato is soft.

2. Place the garlic in a food processor with the S blade inserted. Mince. Add the cooked sweet potato, miso, and tofu. Process until smooth.

3. Return to the soup pot. Stir in the soy milk. Reduce the heat to medium and stir in the dill. Cook until hot. Remove from the heat and stir in the lemon juice. Taste. If needed, add more dill and lemon.

PLANT ESTROGEN ESTIMATE: 1¼ PORTIONS PER SERVING

CORN CHOWDER

Work and Cooking Time: *under 25 minutes*
Equipment: *electric food processor*
Yield: *Makes 4 servings*

The perfect vegetable chowder—creamy, light, protein-packed, and estrogen-enriched. Be careful not to boil—too much heat will make this creamy corn concoction curdle.

Canola-oil spray

1 onion, chopped

6 soy sausages, sliced

2 new potatoes, diced

2 bay leaves

1 cup soy milk

8 ounces frozen corn

2 garlic cloves, quartered

½ cake (9½ ounces) silken tofu

1½ teaspoons dried parsley

Salt and pepper

1. Spray a frying pan with oil. Heat the pan over medium-high heat. Sauté the onion and sausage until the onion is translucent. Set aside.

2. Pour 1 cup of water into a heavy-bottomed soup pot. Add the potatoes. Cook, covered, over high heat until soft. Reduce the heat to medium. Add the potatoes to the sautéed onion and sausage; add the bay leaves, soy milk, and corn.

3. Place the garlic in a food processor with the S blade inserted. Mince. Add the tofu. Process until smooth. Stir the mixture into the soup pot. Add the parsley. Cook until hot, taking care not to boil. Add salt and pepper to taste. Serve.

PLANT ESTROGEN ESTIMATE: 1¼ PORTIONS PER SERVING

TUSCAN BEAN SOUP

Work and Cooking Time: *under 15 minutes*
Equipment: *electric food processor*
Yield: *Makes 4 servings*

A decadent delight designed to add inches to every waistline? This great Italian imitation certainly tastes that good, but it's actually a healthy, high-protein, cream-free food.

Canola-oil spray

4 garlic cloves, sliced

2 onions, chopped

1 cake (16 ounces) soft tofu

½ cup plus ⅔ cup canned cannellini beans

¼ cup fresh parsley

1½ tablespoons dark miso

1 cup soy milk

Pinch pepper

1. Spray a heavy-bottomed soup pot with oil. Sauté the garlic and onion until browned.

2. While the garlic and onion cook, place the tofu, ½ cup of beans, parsley, and miso in a food processor with the S blade inserted. Process for 3 minutes, until smooth.

3. Turn the tofu-bean mixture into the soup pot with the garlic and onion. Immediately whisk in the soy milk. Stir in the ⅔ cup of beans. Add the pepper. Cook over medium heat without boiling. Serve when hot.

PLANT ESTROGEN ESTIMATE: 1¼ PORTIONS PER SERVING

Seven

Condiments

≋ SALTS AND PEPPERS

Put away the salt and pepper shakers. With these salts and peppers, you can shake a little estrogen into every soup, salad, main dish, vegetable, pasta, or grain. You'll add extra taste and cut down on salt at the same time.

SESAME SALT

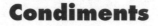

Work Time: *under 3 minutes*
Equipment: *electric coffee grinder*
Yield: *Makes about ⅔ cup*

This Japanese-style condiment will give any meal less salt, more taste, and more essential nutrition.

¼ cup unhulled sesame seeds   1 teaspoon salt
¼ cup flaxseed

Grind the sesame seeds to a coarse texture in an electric coffee grinder. Pour them into a bowl or shaker. Grind the flaxseed to a fine meal. Add to the bowl or shaker. Stir in the salt. Refrigerate between uses.

PLANT ESTROGEN ESTIMATE: **4 PORTIONS PER RECIPE**

FLAX SALT

Work Time: *under 3 minutes*
Equipment: *electric coffee grinder*
Yield: *Makes ½ cup*

Keep this simple salt handy for adding a nutty-salty flavor.

⅓ cup flaxseed
1 teaspoon salt

Place the flaxseed and salt in an electric coffee grinder. Grind to desired texture. Spoon into a cheese shaker. Store in the refrigerator.

PLANT ESTROGEN ESTIMATE: **5 PORTIONS PER RECIPE**

DILL SALT

Work Time: *under 3 minutes*
Equipment: *electric coffee grinder*
Yield: *Makes about ½ cup*

Love the taste of dill? If so, you're in luck: This salt not only gives you plant estrogens, it gives you calcium. Surprised? Did you know dill is a great calcium source? Just shake this concoction on main dishes, soups, and salads for an extra dash of the essential mineral.

¼ cup flaxseed   ½ teaspoon salt
1 tablespoon dill seeds   1 tablespoon dried dill

Place the flaxseed, dill seeds, and salt in an electric coffee grinder. Grind to desired texture. Spoon into a cheese shaker. Stir in the dried dill. Store in the refrigerator.

PLANT ESTROGEN ESTIMATE: 4 PORTIONS PER RECIPE

HERB SALT

Work Time: *under 3 minutes*
Equipment: *electric coffee grinder*
Yield: *Makes about ½ cup*

Feel free to substitute any combination of your favorite dried herbs.

¼ cup flaxseed   1 teaspoon celery seed
1 teaspoon onion powder   1 teaspoon dried parsley
1 teaspoon garlic powder   1 teaspoon dried oregano
1 teaspoon dried tarragon   ½ teaspoon salt

Place the flaxseed in an electric coffee grinder. Grind to desired texture. Pour into a bowl. Stir in the remaining ingredients. Spoon into a cheese shaker. Store in the refrigerator.

PLANT ESTROGEN ESTIMATE: **4** PORTIONS PER RECIPE

CURRY SALT

Work Time: *under 3 minutes*
Equipment: *electric coffee grinder*
Yield: *Makes about ½ cup*

Instantly "curry" your soups, vegetables, and main dishes—just pour on this curry salt.

¼ cup flaxseed
1 teaspoon onion powder
1 teaspoon garlic powder

1 tablespoon curry powder
½ teaspoon salt

Place the flaxseed in an electric coffee grinder. Grind to desired texture. Pour into a bowl. Stir in the remaining ingredients. Spoon into a cheese shaker. Store in the refrigerator.

PLANT ESTROGEN ESTIMATE: **4** PORTIONS PER RECIPE

THAI SALT

Work Time: *under 3 minutes*
Equipment: *electric food processor*
Yield: *Makes about 1 cup*

In Thailand, coarsely ground peanuts with salt get sprinkled on vegetables, fish, and chicken dishes. Use soy nuts to add this Thai touch to food. You'll get less fat and more protein with this estrogenic alternative.

1 cup soy nuts
1 teaspoon salt

Place the soy nuts and salt in a food processor with the S blade inserted. Pulse until coarsely chopped. Spoon into a shaker to serve.

PLANT ESTROGEN ESTIMATE: **4** PORTIONS PER RECIPE

CAJUN PEPPER

Work Time: *under 3 minutes*
Equipment: *electric coffee grinder*
Yield: *Makes about ½ cup*

A mild Cajun pepper to keep you cool. If you like it hot, just substitute cayenne pepper for paprika.

¼ cup flaxseed
1 teaspoon onion powder
1 teaspoon dried thyme

1 tablespoon paprika
1 teaspoon garlic powder
½ teaspoon salt

Place the flaxseed in an electric coffee grinder. Grind to desired texture. Pour into a bowl. Stir in the remaining ingredients. Spoon into a cheese shaker. Store in the refrigerator.

PLANT ESTROGEN ESTIMATE: **4** PORTIONS PER RECIPE

SEEDY PEPPER

Work Time: *under 3 minutes*
Equipment: *electric coffee grinder*
Yield: *Makes about ½ cup*

A simple pepper with added crunch.

¼ cup flaxseed
1 tablespoon black pepper

Place the flaxseed in an electric coffee grinder. Grind to desired texture. Pour into a bowl. Stir in the pepper. Spoon into a cheese shaker. Store in the refrigerator.

PLANT ESTROGEN ESTIMATE: **4** PORTIONS PER RECIPE

CRUNCHY PAPRIKA

Work Time: *under 3 minutes*
Equipment: *electric coffee grinder*
Yield: *Makes about ½ cup*

A bright-red two-ingredient recipe! Sprinkle on color, flavor, and plant estrogens.

¼ cup flaxseed
1 tablespoon paprika

Place the flaxseed in an electric coffee grinder. Grind to desired texture. Pour into a bowl. Stir in the paprika. Spoon into a cheese shaker. Store in the refrigerator.

PLANT ESTROGEN ESTIMATE: **4 PORTIONS PER RECIPE**

≋ SEASONING SAUCES

Barbecue, curry, teriyaki, satay—sauces make any boring grain, vegetable, fish, or poultry dish interesting. Most seasoning sauces use lots of oil or cream. With tofu, you don't need either.

CURRY SAUCE

Work Time: *under 5 minutes*
Yield: *Makes 1 cup*

A subtly sweet and salty curry sauce—great with fish or poultry.

1 tablespoon curry powder
1 teaspoon ground cinnamon
1 teaspoon tamari
2 garlic cloves, minced

¼ cup frozen apple juice concentrate
1 cup soy milk
¼ cake (4¾ ounces) silken tofu

Whisk together all of the ingredients until thickened. Serve.

PLANT ESTROGEN ESTIMATE: **2 PORTIONS PER RECIPE**

GINGER SOY SAUCE

Work Time: *under 5 minutes*
Equipment: *electric blender*
Yield: *Makes 1 cup*

This sauce, with its Chinese flavor, will dress up vegetables and grains.

2 tablespoons tamari
2 teaspoons grated fresh ginger

2 garlic cloves, minced
2 tablespoons flaxseed

Place all of the ingredients and 1 cup of water in an electric blender. Blend until smooth.

PLANT ESTROGEN ESTIMATE: 1½ PORTIONS PER RECIPE

LIGHTLY CREAMY GINGER SAUCE

Work Time: *under 5 minutes*
Equipment: *electric blender*
Yield: *Makes about 1 cup*

Add flavor to grains, vegetables, even fish or poultry dishes, with this simple sauce.

1 tablespoon grated fresh ginger
2 garlic cloves, pressed
2 tablespoons tamari

¾ cup unsweetened soy milk
¼ cake (4¾ ounces) silken tofu

Place all of the ingredients in an electric blender. Blend until smooth. Refrigerate between servings.

PLANT ESTROGEN ESTIMATE: 1¾ PORTIONS PER RECIPE

TAHINI SAUCE

Work Time: *under 5 minutes*
Equipment: *electric blender*
Yield: *Makes 1 cup*

A Middle Eastern flavor—the perfect sauce for falafel.

1½ tablespoons tahini
1 tablespoon lemon juice
2 garlic cloves, minced

1 cup unsweetened soy milk
¼ cake (4¾ ounces) silken tofu
Salt

Place the tahini, lemon juice, garlic, soy milk, and tofu in an electric blender. Blend until smooth. Salt to taste. Serve.

PLANT ESTROGEN ESTIMATE: **2** PORTIONS PER RECIPE

CREAMY SATAY SAUCE

Work Time: *under 5 minutes*
Equipment: *electric blender*
Yield: *Makes 1 cup*

This Thai-style peanut sauce works well with grilled chicken, tofu, or vegetables.

2 tablespoons peanut butter
1 tablespoon soy sauce
2 garlic cloves, minced

1 cup unsweetened soy milk
¼ cake (4¾ ounces) silken tofu

Place all of the ingredients in an electric blender. Blend until smooth. Serve.

PLANT ESTROGEN ESTIMATE: **2** PORTIONS PER RECIPE

GUILT-FREE GRAVY

Work and Cooking Time: *under 5 minutes*
Equipment: *electric food processor*
Yield: *Makes about 1½ cups*

From mashed potatoes to sliced turkey, use this gravy without guilt. When you indulge, you pour on protein, calcium, and plant estrogens.

And this gravy is foolproof—it's as creamy as a white-flour gravy, but it never has lumps.

2 garlic cloves, quartered
1 teaspoon tahini
¾ cup unsweetened soy milk

½ cake (9½ ounces) silken tofu
1 tablespoon tamari

Place the garlic in a food processor with the S blade inserted. Process until minced. Add the remaining ingredients. Process until smooth. Taste. If needed, add more tamari. Pour into a saucepan. Heat over medium-high heat until hot. Serve.

PLANT ESTROGEN ESTIMATE: **2** PORTIONS PER RECIPE

GARLIC SOUR CREME

Work Time: *under 5 minutes*
Equipment: *electric food processor*
Yield: *Makes about 1 cup*

Do you crave sour cream? Try this naturally estrogenic creamy garlic sauce instead.

2 garlic cloves, quartered
1 tablespoon lemon juice
½ cake (8 ounces) soft tofu

Salt
3 tablespoons finely chopped chives

Place the garlic in a food processor with the S blade inserted. Process until minced. Add the lemon juice and tofu. Process for 2 minutes, until smooth and silky. Salt to taste. Turn into a bowl. Stir in the chives. Refrigerate between servings.

PLANT ESTROGEN ESTIMATE: **2** PORTIONS PER RECIPE

Eight

Salads and Side Dishes

Let's face it: Soybeans and flaxseeds are just too drab. Look at them. You'll see a full spectrum from beige to brown. Vegetables and fruits are different. Green, orange, yellow, pink, purple, and red—they're just too pretty not to be good. Not only do they add color and crunch to eating, they may just give an extra boost to your estrogen intake. Vegetables and fruits are among the best sources of the mineral boron. People are talking a lot about and making big claims for the positive effects of boron on estrogen and calcium. Dr. Forrest Neilson, the man who did most of the research, isn't proclaiming boron the miracle menopausal cure. Instead, he's cautious. He has noticed that under certain conditions, with the help of other nutrients (he's not entirely sure which ones), boron does indeed appear to elevate estrogen levels and decrease calcium loss. Certainly all the many vitamins and minerals packed in lovely, crispy vegetables and fruits make them essential edibles for staying vibrant.

CREAMY DILL VINAIGRETTE

≋

Work Time: *under 5 minutes*
Equipment: *electric food processor*
Yield: *Makes about 1 cup*

Go heavy on the dill; don't skimp on the garlic.

3 garlic cloves, quartered	½ cup soy milk
½ cake (9½ ounces) silken tofu	2 tablespoons snipped fresh dill
1 teaspoon Dijon mustard	Salt
2 tablespoons vinegar	

Place the garlic in a food processor with the S blade inserted. Mince. Add the remaining ingredients and process until smooth and silky. Taste. Add more salt and dill if needed. Pour into a bottle. Refrigerate between servings.

PLANT ESTROGEN ESTIMATE: **2½** PORTIONS PER RECIPE

TOMATO-BACIN DRESSING

≋

Work Time: *under 5 minutes*
Equipment: *electric food processor*
Yield: *Makes about 1¼ cups*

You can find all-natural bacin bits. They add a bit of soy and a lot of flavor.

2 garlic cloves, quartered	2 tablespoons vinegar
1 cup canned diced tomatoes in juice	3 tablespoons bacin bits
¼ cake (4½ ounces) silken tofu	Salt

Place the garlic in a food processor with the S blade inserted. Mince. Add the tomatoes with their juice, tofu, vinegar, and bacin bits. Process until puréed. Salt to taste. Pour into a bottle. Refrigerate between servings.

PLANT ESTROGEN ESTIMATE: **1** PORTION PER RECIPE

ROASTED RED PEPPER-AND-OLIVE DRESSING

Work Time: *under 5 minutes*
Equipment: *electric food processor*
Yield: *Makes about 1 cup*

Bright red with black bits, this dressing adds festive color to any green salad.

2 garlic cloves, quartered
¾ cup (7 ounces) bottled roasted red peppers, drained
2 tablespoons high-lignan flax oil

¼ cake (4½ ounces) silken tofu
3 tablespoons pitted Greek olives
Salt

Place the garlic in a food processor with the S blade inserted. Mince. Add the peppers, oil, and tofu. Process until puréed. Add the olives. Pulse several times to chop the olives. Salt to taste. Pour into a bottle. Refrigerate between servings.

PLANT ESTROGEN ESTIMATE: **1** PORTION PER RECIPE

CREAMY SESAME DRESSING

Work Time: *under 5 minutes*
Equipment: *electric blender*
Yield: *Makes about 1 cup*

If you love the taste of sesame, this dressing will be a favorite.

½ cake (9½ ounces) silken tofu
⅔ cup soy milk

1½ tablespoons tamari
1 tablespoon tahini

Place all of the ingredients in an electric blender. Blend until smooth. Pour into a bottle. Refrigerate between servings.

PLANT ESTROGEN ESTIMATE: 2⅔ PORTIONS PER RECIPE

LIGHTLY CREAMY DIJON VINAIGRETTE

Work Time: *under 5 minutes*
Equipment: *electric blender*
Yield: *Makes about 1 cup*

Quick and easy—a basic, everyday dressing.

1 garlic clove, pressed
1 tablespoon Dijon mustard
1 tablespoon apple cider vinegar

¼ cake (4¾ ounces) silken tofu
½ cup soy milk
Salt

Place the garlic, mustard, vinegar, tofu, and soy milk in an electric blender. Blend until fully mixed. Salt to taste. Pour into a bottle. Refrigerate between servings.

PLANT ESTROGEN ESTIMATE: 1½ PORTIONS PER SERVING

FRESH BASIL DRESSING

Work Time: *under 5 minutes*
Equipment: *electric food processor*
Yield: *Makes about ¾ cup*

Add some of this fresh green dressing to your fresh green salad.

2 garlic cloves, quartered

½ cup fresh basil leaves

¼ cake (4¾ ounces) silken tofu

½ cup unsweetened soy milk

1 teaspoon apple cider vinegar

Salt

Place the garlic in a food processor with the S blade inserted. Mince. Add the basil, tofu, soy milk, and vinegar. Process until puréed. Salt to taste. Pour into a bottle. Refrigerate between servings.

PLANT ESTROGEN ESTIMATE: 1½ PORTIONS PER RECIPE

AVOCADO-CILANTRO DRESSING

Work Time: *under 5 minutes*
Equipment: *electric food processor*
Yield: *Makes about 1 cup*

How can an avocado dressing be bad?

2 garlic cloves, quartered

¼ cup fresh cilantro leaves

1 avocado, peeled and sliced

¼ cake (4 ounces) soft tofu

½ cup soy milk

1 tablespoon lemon juice

Salt

Place the garlic in a food processor with the S blade inserted. Mince. Add the cilantro and chop. Add the avocado, tofu, soy milk, and lemon juice. Process for 2 minutes, until smooth. Salt to taste. Pour into a bottle. Refrigerate between servings.

PLANT ESTROGEN ESTIMATE: **3** PORTIONS PER RECIPE

SWEET ORANGE DRESSING

Work Time: *under 5 minutes*
Equipment: *electric blender*
Yield: *Makes about ¾ cup*

Try this dressing tossed with grated carrots, spooned over chopped apples and raisins, or as a sauce for fruit salad.

½ cake (9½ ounces) silken tofu
2 tablespoons frozen orange juice concentrate
1 teaspoon grated orange rind

1 tablespoon apple cider vinegar
Salt

Place the tofu, orange juice concentrate, orange rind, and vinegar in an electric blender. Blend until smooth. Salt to taste. Pour into a bottle. Refrigerate between servings.

PLANT ESTROGEN ESTIMATE: **2** PORTIONS PER RECIPE

LEMON-FLAXSEED SALAD DRESSING

Work Time: *under 5 minutes*
Yield: *Makes 1¼ cups*

A lightly creamy dressing with a bit of crunch.

2 garlic cloves, pressed

2 tablespoons lemon juice

3 tablespoons high-lignan flax oil

2 tablespoons tamari

2 tablespoons flaxseed

1 cup unsweetened soy milk

Place the garlic, lemon juice, flax oil, tamari, and flaxseed in a small mixing bowl. Mix until well combined. Add the soy milk. Whip with a wire whisk until well combined.

PLANT ESTROGEN ESTIMATE: 3½ PORTIONS PER RECIPE

MUSTARD VINAIGRETTE

Work Time: *under 5 minutes*
Yield: *Makes ¾ cup*

A vinaigrette with a tangy mustard taste.

1 tablespoon vinegar

1 tablespoon tamari

½ cup unsweetened soy milk

2 tablespoons flaxseed

2 tablespoons high-lignan flax oil

1 tablespoon Dijon mustard

Place all of the ingredients in a small mixing bowl. Whip with a wire whisk until well combined.

PLANT ESTROGEN ESTIMATE: 2¾ PORTIONS PER RECIPE

HERB VINAIGRETTE

Work Time: *under 5 minutes*
Yield: *Makes ½ cup*

This combination of herbs lends added flavor to any green salad.

2 tablespoons vinegar
1 tablespoon tamari
½ cup unsweetened soy milk
1 teaspoon dried parsley

1 teaspoon dried dill
½ teaspoon dried oregano
1 tablespoon flaxseed
3 tablespoons high-lignan flax oil

Place all of the ingredients in a small mixing bowl. Whip with a wire whisk until well combined. Spoon over green salad. Toss.

PLANT ESTROGEN ESTIMATE: **2** PORTIONS PER RECIPE

SALADS

These salads don't provide large quantities of plant estrogen, but they all bring balance to a healthy diet.

POTATO SALAD

Work and Cooking Time: *under 20 minutes*
Waiting Time: *30 minutes*
Equipment: *electric food processor*
Yield: *Makes 4 servings*

A hearty, high-protein version of a summertime staple. Be sure to rinse and cool the potatoes. If you add the dressing while the potatoes are hot, the dressing cooks—it gets thicker and thicker.

4 new potatoes, halved	¼ teaspoon salt
4 garlic cloves, quartered	1 cake (16 ounces) soft tofu
1 tablespoon snipped fresh dill	1 onion, chopped
2 tablespoons apple cider vinegar	1 cup chopped dill pickles
3 tablespoons Dijon mustard	

1. Place the potatoes in a cooking pot; cover with water. Boil until the potatoes can be pierced with a knife. Remove from the heat. Rinse with cool water. Place in the refrigerator to cool.

2. Place the garlic in a food processor with the S blade inserted. Mince. Add the dill, vinegar, mustard, salt, and tofu. Process until smooth. Pour into a salad bowl.

3. Add the onion and pickles. Cut the cooled potatoes into ½-inch cubes. Add. Fold all of the ingredients together until thoroughly combined. Serve.

PLANT ESTROGEN ESTIMATE: 1 PORTION PER SERVING

WATERCRESS, ROMAINE, AND WALNUT SALAD

Work Time: *under 10 minutes*
Equipment: *electric food processor*
Yield: *Makes 4 servings*

Try to find young, small watercress leaves for this salad.

1 medium head romaine	2 garlic cloves, quartered
1 cup young watercress	½ cake (8 ounces) soft tofu
½ cup coarsely chopped walnuts	2 tablespoons apple cider vinegar
Salt	2 tablespoons frozen apple juice concentrate

1. Tear the romaine and place it in a bowl. Add the watercress (if necessary, remove the stems) and walnuts. Lightly salt and toss.

2. Place the garlic in a food processor with the S blade inserted. Mince. Add the tofu, vinegar, and apple juice concentrate. Process until smooth. Pour over the greens and walnuts and toss well.

PLANT ESTROGEN ESTIMATE: ½ PORTION PER SERVING

AVOCADO WITH GREENS

Work Time: *under 10 minutes*
Equipment: *electric food processor*
Yield: *Makes 4 servings*

Green, purple, and orange—great colors tossed in a creamy avocado dressing.

½ large head romaine	2 garlic cloves, quartered
½ small head radicchio	1 large ripe avocado, peeled and sliced
1 carrot	1 tablespoon apple cider vinegar
Salt	¼ cake (4¾ ounces) silken tofu

1. Tear the romaine and radicchio into bite-size pieces and place in a salad bowl. Grate the carrot into the bowl. Salt and toss.

2. Place the garlic in a food processor with the S blade inserted. Mince. Add the remaining ingredients. Process until smooth. Pour over the salad. Toss and serve.

PLANT ESTROGEN ESTIMATE: ¼ PORTION PER SERVING

ANISE-AND-APPLE WALDORF SALAD

Work Time: *under 15 minutes*
Equipment: *electric food processor*
Yield: *Makes 4 servings*

Give Waldorf salad a taste twist—use fresh anise instead of celery. I've read that anise has estrogenic qualities, but I have no idea how much.

½ cup chopped walnuts
1 medium bulb fresh anise, chopped
3 sweet apples, chopped
½ cake (8 ounces) soft tofu

2 tablespoons frozen apple juice concentrate
1 teaspoon lemon juice
½ teaspoon anise extract

1. Place the walnuts, anise, and apples in a salad bowl.
2. Place the tofu, apple juice concentrate, lemon juice, and anise extract in a food processor with the S blade inserted. Process for 2 minutes, until smooth and silky.
3. Fold the tofu mixture into the chopped nuts, anise, and apples. Mix thoroughly.

PLANT ESTROGEN ESTIMATE: ½ PORTION PER SERVING

SPINACH-SESAME SALAD

Work Time: *under 15 minutes*
Yield: *Makes 2 servings*

This Japanese-style side dish is packed with calcium, iron, natural estrogen, and omega-3s.

¼ cake (4 ounces) extra-firm tofu
2 garlic cloves, pressed
1 teaspoon tamari
10 ounces fresh spinach, steamed

1 teaspoon rice vinegar
2 tablespoons high-lignan flax oil
2 tablespoons sesame seeds

1. Place the tofu, garlic, and tamari in a medium-size bowl. Mash together with a fork, combining thoroughly.

2. Add the spinach. Toss until the tofu mixture is thoroughly combined with the spinach. Add the vinegar and toss. Add the oil and toss. Add the sesame seeds and toss.

PLANT ESTROGEN ESTIMATE: ⅔ PORTION PER SERVING

TOMATOES WITH FRESH BASIL MARINADE

Work Time: *under 15 minutes*
Yield: *Makes 4 servings*

A pretty arrangement of tomatoes with a fresh basil topping. This is a wonderfully simple way to use fresh summer food and increase your natural estrogen intake.

3 tomatoes, sliced
1 small onion, chopped fine
1 garlic clove, minced
2 tablespoons chopped fresh basil

1 tablespoon balsamic vinegar
2 tablespoons high-lignan flax oil
¼ cake (4 ounces) extra-firm tofu
Salt

1. Arrange the sliced tomatoes in concentric circles on a dinner plate.

2. Place the onion, garlic, basil, vinegar, oil, and tofu in a small mixing bowl. Mash with a fork or potato masher until thoroughly combined. Salt to taste. Spoon over the tomatoes.

PLANT ESTROGEN ESTIMATE: ⅓ PORTION PER SERVING

NUTTY ORANGE-CARROT SALAD

Work Time: *under 10 minutes*
Yield: *Makes 4 servings*

This sweet-and-sour grated carrot salad with nuts is a simple estrogenic addition to any season.

5 carrots, grated	2 tablespoons high-lignan flax oil
Salt	¼ cup raisins
1 tablespoon frozen orange juice concentrate	½ cup soy nuts
1 tablespoon frozen apple juice concentrate	

Place the grated carrot in a salad bowl. Sprinkle with salt and toss. Add the orange juice concentrate and toss. Add the apple juice concentrate and toss. Add the flax oil and toss. Mix in the raisins and soy nuts.

PLANT ESTROGEN ESTIMATE: ½ PORTION PER SERVING

CREAMY CRANBERRY SALAD

Work and Cooking Time: *under 10 minutes*
Chilling Time: *2 hours*
Equipment: *electric food processor*
Yield: *Makes 6 servings*

Crunchy nuts and melt-in-your-mouth creaminess in shades of pink. At our family's Thanksgiving dinners, this festive dish disappears first.

¾ cup frozen apple juice concentrate, thawed
1 envelope (1 tablespoon) unflavored gelatin
½ cup chopped walnuts
12 ounces fresh cranberries, chopped

½ cake (9½ ounces) silken tofu
¼ cup raw sugar or maple syrup
½ teaspoon ground cardamom

1. Place ¼ cup of the apple juice concentrate in a small bowl. Sprinkle the gelatin over the surface. Pour the remaining ½ cup of concentrate into a saucepan. Heat over medium-high heat. When the gelatin has dissolved, stir it into the heated juice. Continue to simmer.

2. Place the walnuts and cranberries in a medium-size mixing bowl. Stir in the gelatin–and–apple juice concentrate mixture.

3. Place the tofu, sugar, and cardamom in a food processor with the S blade inserted. Process until smooth and silky. Fold into the cranberry mixture. Turn into a serving bowl or gelatin mold. Chill until firm. Unmold before serving.

PLANT ESTROGEN ESTIMATE: ⅓ PORTION PER SERVING

ISRAELI SALAD

Work Time: *under 15 minutes*
Yield: *Makes 4 servings*

In Israel, you can eat this combination of fresh summer vegetables at any time of day— even for breakfast. Substituting caper-and-olive-flavored tofu for feta, and flax oil for olive oil, changes the tradition. Now, it's naturally estrogenic.

2 tomatoes, cut into 1-inch chunks
1 medium cucumber, sliced
1 green bell pepper, cut into 1-inch chunks
2 garlic cloves, minced
¼ cup pitted Greek olives, chopped fine

1 tablespoon capers, chopped fine
½ cake (8 ounces) extra-firm tofu
1 tablespoon vinegar
3 tablespoons high-lignan flax oil

1. Place the tomatoes, cucumber, and green pepper in a salad bowl.

2. Place the garlic, olives, capers, and tofu in a mixing bowl. Mash until all are thoroughly combined. Spoon over the vegetables and toss. Add the vinegar and toss. Add the flax oil and toss.

PLANT ESTROGEN ESTIMATE: ¾ PORTION PER SERVING

CUCUMBER-BASIL SALAD

Work Time: *under 10 minutes*
Equipment: *electric food processor*
Yield: *Makes 2 servings*

A creamy summer salad in shades of green.

2 garlic cloves, quartered
½ cake (9½ ounces) silken tofu
1 cup fresh basil

1 tablespoon apple cider vinegar
Salt
1 large English cucumber, sliced

1. Place the garlic in a food processor with the S blade inserted. Mince. Add the tofu, basil, and vinegar. Process until smooth. Salt to taste.

2. Slice the cucumber. Place in a salad bowl. Add the tofu purée and stir in. Serve.

PLANT ESTROGEN ESTIMATE: 1 PORTION PER SERVING

How can you put a little plant estrogen in your hot veggies? Three ways:

1. Creamy sauces
2. Tasty glazes
3. Brightly colored loaves

You'll find all three in these side dish recipes.

HOT ARTICHOKES IN LEMON SAUCE

≋

Work and Cooking Time: *under 10 minutes*
Equipment: *electric food processor*
Yield: *Makes 6 servings*

Tastes rich. Feels like massive amounts of calories. Not true! It's a low-fat side dish to delight the gourmet in you. You can use canned or frozen artichoke hearts. In this dish, I actually prefer the taste of canned!

Take care. If you mix in the lemon while the artichokes and sauce are still cooking, the mixture will curdle.

4 garlic cloves, quartered	1 pound artichoke hearts, canned or frozen
2 tablespoons capers	3 tablespoons lemon juice
1 cake (about 19 ounces) silken tofu	Salt

1. Place the garlic in a food processor with the S blade inserted. Mince. Add the capers and tofu. Process until smooth.

2. Pour the tofu mixture into a saucepan. Add the drained or thawed artichokes. Cook over medium heat without boiling until fully heated. Remove from the burner.

Add the lemon juice. Stir. Salt to taste. Taste again. If needed, add more lemon juice and salt. Serve.

PLANT ESTROGEN ESTIMATE: ⅔ PORTION PER SERVING

PEA PODS, CARROTS, AND NUTS
IN SWEET GINGER GLAZE

Work and Cooking Time: *20 minutes*
Yield: *Makes 4 servings*

This bright orange-and-green dish has a delicately sweet and nearly invisible glaze.

3 carrots, sliced
⅔ cup apple juice
8 ⅛×1-inch slices fresh ginger
2 teaspoons cornstarch

1 tablespoon frozen apple juice concentrate
1 tablespoon high-lignan flax oil
1 cup fresh pea pods
½ cup soy nuts

1. Steam the carrots over 2 cups of water for 5 minutes or until tender.

2. While the carrots steam, prepare the glaze: Pour the apple juice into a pan. Add the ginger. Simmer for 10 minutes. Dissolve the cornstarch in the apple juice concentrate. Stir into the cooking juice and ginger. Continue stirring until the glaze thickens. Remove from the heat. Whisk in the oil.

3. Place the pea pods in boiling water for no longer than 1 minute, until bright green.

4. Combine the carrots and pea pods in a bowl. Pour the ginger glaze over them. Toss. Sprinkle on soy nuts. Serve.

PLANT ESTROGEN ESTIMATE: ½ PORTION PER SERVING

CARROT AND ANISE IN CREAMY SAUCE

Work and Cooking Time: *under 15 minutes*
Equipment: *electric food processor*
Yield: *Makes 4 servings*

Michael says this is too good to be a vegetable dish. His suggestion: "Put it on pasta. It's great. It should be a main dish."

If you've never eaten anise, this combination of carrots and anise in a light, delicious sauce is a good place to start.

Canola-oil spray
3 garlic cloves, minced
1 onion, chopped
3 carrots, sliced
1 medium anise bulb, sliced

1 cup soy milk
½ cake (9½ ounces) silken tofu
¼ teaspoon anise extract
Salt and pepper

1. Spray a heavy frying pan with oil. Heat the pan over medium-high heat. Sauté the garlic, onion, and carrot until the carrot can be pierced with a fork. Add the anise. Continue cooking until the carrot is tender and the anise can be pierced with a fork.

2. While the vegetables cook, prepare the sauce: Place the soy milk, tofu, and anise extract in a food processor with the S blade inserted. Process until smooth and silky.

3. Pour the sauce over the vegetables. Continue cooking without boiling until the sauce is heated. Add salt and pepper to taste. Serve.

PLANT ESTROGEN ESTIMATE: ½ PORTION PER SERVING

GREEN BEANS, SUN-DRIED TOMATOES, AND WALNUTS

Work and Cooking Time: *under 15 minutes*
Yield: *Makes 4 servings*

1 pound green beans
¼ cup minced bottled sun-dried tomatoes
2 garlic cloves, pressed
⅓ cup chopped walnuts

2 teaspoons apple cider vinegar
1 tablespoon high-lignan flax oil
½ cake (8 ounces) extra-firm tofu

1. Steam the green beans over 2 cups of water for 5 minutes or until tender.
2. Combine the sun-dried tomatoes, garlic, walnuts, vinegar, and oil in a salad bowl. Mash in the tofu. Add the prepared beans. Toss.

PLANT ESTROGEN ESTIMATE: ½ PORTION PER SERVING

ASPARAGUS WITH LEMON-GARLIC SAUCE

Work and Cooking Time: *under 10 minutes*
Equipment: *electric food processor*
Yield: *Makes 4 servings*

A simply delicious way to serve fresh asparagus—all the creaminess, none of the cholesterol.

3 garlic cloves, quartered
½ cake (9½ ounces) silken tofu
3 tablespoons lemon juice

¼ cup chopped scallion
Salt
1 pound fresh asparagus

1. Place the garlic in a food processor with the S blade inserted. Mince. Add the tofu, lemon juice, and scallion. Process until smooth. Salt to taste. Taste again. If needed, add more lemon juice.

2. Steam the asparagus for 3 to 5 minutes, just until bright green. Place on a serving plate. Spoon the lemon sauce over the asparagus. Serve.

PLANT ESTROGEN ESTIMATE: ½ PORTION PER SERVING

MINI CARROT LOAVES

Work and Cooking Time: *under 15 minutes*
Baking Time: *20 minutes*
Equipment: *electric food processor*
Yield: *Makes 4 servings*

A small, sweet, bright-orange vegetable loaf.

2 cups sliced carrots
3 garlic cloves, quartered
4 ⅛×1-inch slices fresh ginger

1 cake (16 ounces) firm tofu
1 tablespoon yellow miso

1. Preheat the oven to 350°F.

2. Steam the carrots over 2 cups of water for 5 minutes or until tender.

3. Place the garlic and ginger in a food processor with the S blade inserted. Mince. Break the tofu into several smaller chunks. Place them in the processor. Add the yellow miso. Process until smooth. Add the steamed carrots. Process until fully combined.

4. Turn the mixture into four nonstick or oiled 4½-inch tart pans or four muffin tins. Bake for 20 minutes, until firm and lightly browned. Remove from the pans to serve.

PLANT ESTROGEN ESTIMATE: 1 PORTION PER SERVING

MINI SPINACH LOAVES

Work and Cooking Time: *under 15 minutes*
Baking Time: *20 minutes*
Equipment: *electric food processor*
Yield: *Makes 4 servings*

A festive way to eat your spinach.

20 ounces fresh spinach

4 garlic cloves, quartered

4 ⅛×1-inch slices fresh ginger

1 cake (16 ounces) firm tofu

Salt

1. Preheat the oven to 350°F.

2. Steam the spinach over 2 cups of water for 5 minutes or until tender.

3. Place the garlic and ginger in a food processor with the S blade inserted. Mince. Break the tofu into several smaller chunks. Place them in the processor. Process until smooth. Add the steamed spinach. Process until fully combined. Salt to taste.

4. Turn the mixture into four nonstick or oiled 4½-inch tart pans or four muffin tins. Bake for 20 minutes, until firm and lightly browned. Remove from the pans to serve.

PLANT ESTROGEN ESTIMATE: **1** PORTION PER SERVING

ORANGE AND GREEN PÂTÉ

Work and Cooking Time: *under 20 minutes*
Baking Time: *30 minutes*
Equipment: *electric food processor*
Yield: *Makes 8 servings*

Want a dish to awaken admiration? Try this one. Its bright green-and-orange stripes are sure to impress.

Orange layers
2 cups sliced carrots
3 garlic cloves, quartered
4 ⅛×1-inch slices fresh ginger
1 cake (16 ounces) firm tofu
1 tablespoon yellow miso

Green layers
20 ounces fresh spinach
4 garlic cloves, quartered
4 ⅛×1-inch slices fresh ginger
1 cake (16 ounces) firm tofu
1 tablespoon yellow miso

1. Preheat the oven to 350°F.

2. Prepare the carrot pâté: Steam the carrots over 2 cups of water for 5 minutes or until tender. Place the garlic and ginger in a food processor with the S blade inserted. Mince. Break the tofu into several smaller chunks. Place them in the processor. Add the yellow miso. Process until smooth. Add the steamed carrots. Process until fully combined. Taste. If needed, add more miso. Turn the mixture into a bowl.

3. Prepare the spinach pâté: Steam the spinach over 2 cups of water for 5 minutes or until tender. Place the garlic and ginger in the processor. Mince. Break the tofu into several smaller chunks. Place them in the processor. Add the yellow miso. Process until smooth. Add the steamed spinach. Process until fully combined. Taste. If needed, add more miso.

4. Spread half the carrot pâté in a 9×5-inch nonstick or oiled loaf pan. Spread half the spinach pâté on top. Use the remainder of the carrot pâté to make another layer. Use the remainder of the spinach pâté to make a final layer.

5. Bake for 30 minutes, until firm and lightly browned. Remove from the pan by covering with a serving plate, then turning over. Serve.

PLANT ESTROGEN ESTIMATE: 1 PORTION PER SERVING

CREAMED POTATOES

Work and Cooking Time: *under 20 minutes*
Equipment: *electric food processor*
Yield: *Makes 4 servings*

A nutritionally rich, creamy sauce. This potato dish provides enough protein to be served as a main dish.

4 potatoes, peeled and sliced thin
Spray oil
1 large onion, sliced thin
3 garlic cloves, quartered
¼ cup fresh parsley

1 tablespoon powdered vegetable soup stock
¼ teaspoon black pepper
½ cup unsweetened soy milk
1 cake (19 ounces) silken tofu

1. Place the potatoes in a cooking pot. Cover with water. Bring to a boil. Simmer until fully cooked. Drain.

2. While the potatoes cook, prepare the cream sauce: Spray a heavy frying pan with oil. Sauté the onion over medium-high heat until translucent. Reduce the heat to low.

3. Place the garlic in a food processor with the S blade inserted. Mince. Add the parsley, soup stock, pepper, soy milk, and tofu. Process until smooth. Add to the onion. Heat without boiling. Stir in the potatoes. Serve.

PLANT ESTROGEN ESTIMATE: 1½ PORTIONS PER SERVING

POTATO LATKES

Work Time: *under 20 minutes*
Baking Time: *15 minutes*
Equipment: *electric food processor*
Yield: *Makes 4 servings*

Latkes don't have to drown in oil to be crispy. At our house, these oven-baked, naturally estrogenic, protein-packed potato pancakes have replaced their fat-filled predecessors. Now, we eat these family favorites to our heart's content.

There's an additional plus: These goodies can be baked in large numbers on cookie sheets. You can serve them in one large, crispy batch. Gone are the days when you stood watch over a frying pan of boiling oil while others ate.

4 large potatoes
3 medium onions
1 cake (16 ounces) soft tofu

Salt and pepper
Spray oil

1. Preheat the oven to 500°F.

2. Alternate grating half a potato and half an onion, using the grating blade of a food processor. (By alternating the potato and onion, the onion juice keeps the potato from discoloring.) Remove from the food processor and place in a mixing bowl.

3. Place the tofu in the food processor with the S blade inserted. Process until smooth. Add to the potato-and-onion mixture, and fold in. Add salt and pepper to taste.

4. Form pancakes by taking large spoonfuls of the latke mixture, placing them on a cookie sheet, and flattening them. Spray the latkes with oil. Turn the latkes over and spray the other sides with oil.

5. Bake for about 5 minutes, until the undersides are lightly browned. Turn the latkes over and bake them until the bottoms are browned and the latkes are crisp.

PLANT ESTROGEN ESTIMATE: **1** PORTION PER SERVING

CREAMED CORN

Work and Cooking Time: *under 10 minutes*
Equipment: *electric food processor*
Yield: *Makes 4 servings*

A recipe for homemade creamy corn that reminds me of a childhood favorite—the canned kind.

2 garlic cloves, quartered
¼ onion, quartered
1 cake (19 ounces) silken tofu
2 pinches turmeric
1 tablespoon frozen white grape juice
    concentrate

Salt
1 pound fresh corn kernels or frozen corn,
    thawed

1. Place the garlic in a food processor with the S blade inserted. Mince. Add the onion. Chop. Add the tofu, turmeric, and juice concentrate. Process until smooth. Salt to taste.

2. Add the corn. Pulse until about half the kernels are chopped and half remain whole. Pour into a saucepan. Heat. Serve.

PLANT ESTROGEN ESTIMATE: 1 PORTION PER SERVING

Nine

Pasta and Rice

All the dishes in this chapter come with added plant estrogens. As a bonus, each recipe brings you precious omega-3 essential fatty acids or additional protein. All make your meal more nutritionally complete.

≋ PASTA WITH TOSSING SAUCES

Mash tofu with irresistible tastes—roasted red peppers, fresh basil, sun-dried tomatoes—and it's transformed into an appealing sauce. Toss it with pasta and you have a dish permeated with protein and impregnated with plant estrogens.

EGGPLANT AND PENNE IN RED PEPPER SAUCE

Work and Cooking Time: *20 minutes*
Equipment: *electric food processor*
Yield: *Makes 4 servings*

A delicious one-dish meal that's a summertime favorite.

1 eggplant, sliced

8 ounces penne

3 garlic cloves, quartered

1 cup fresh basil

12-ounce jar roasted red peppers, drained

1 cake (16 ounces) extra-firm tofu

2 tablespoons balsamic vinegar

Salt

1. Preheat the broiler.

2. Place the sliced eggplant under the broiler. Broil for 5 minutes. Turn over. Broil for 5 more minutes, until browned. Remove from the broiler. When cool enough to touch, cut into ¼-inch strips.

3. Bring 3 quarts of water to a boil. Add the penne and cook for 10 minutes (or according to package directions).

4. While the pasta cooks, prepare the sauce: Place the garlic in a food processor with the S blade inserted. Mince. Add the basil. Mince. Add the drained red peppers. Purée. Pour into a large pasta bowl. Add the tofu. Mash with a potato masher or fork. Add the eggplant and drained pasta. Toss. Add the vinegar and toss. Salt to taste and serve.

> **PLANT ESTROGEN ESTIMATE: 1 PORTION PER SERVING**

SUN-DRIED TOMATO AND
WALNUT TOSS WITH PENNE

Work and Cooking Time: *under 15 minutes*
Yield: *Makes 4 servings*

This recipe is equally appealing served hot or cold.

As is, this recipe makes a great side dish. To make it into a one-dish meal, add your favorite steamed vegetables—asparagus, artichoke hearts, pea pods, and/or green beans.

8 ounces penne

4 garlic cloves, pressed

⅓ cup chopped walnuts

¾ cup minced bottled sun-dried tomatoes

2 tablespoon high-lignan flax oil

1 tablespoon dried basil

½ cake (8 ounces) extra-firm tofu

Salt

1. Bring 3 quarts of water to a boil. Add the penne and cook for 10 minutes (or according to package directions).

2. While the pasta cooks, prepare the sauce: Place the pressed garlic in a large bowl. Add the walnuts, sun-dried tomatoes, oil, and basil. Mash in the tofu and mix well with a spoon.

3. When the penne is ready, drain it and add it to the large bowl. Toss all of the ingredients until pasta is well coated. Pour onto a platter and serve hot or cold.

PLANT ESTROGEN ESTIMATE: ½ **PORTION PER SERVING**

ORZO WITH ROASTED RED
PEPPER-AND-WATERCRESS SAUCE

Work and Cooking Time: *under 15 minutes*
Equipment: *electric food processor*
Yield: *Makes 4 servings*

The bright red-and-green sauce makes this a festive dish.

⅔ cup orzo

3 garlic cloves, quartered

7-ounce jar roasted red peppers, drained

1 cake (16 ounces) extra-firm tofu

2 tablespoons capers

1 cup young watercress (about 1½ inches
   long, including stems)

1. Bring 2 quarts of water to a boil. Add the orzo and cook for 6 to 8 minutes (or according to package directions).

2. While the orzo cooks, prepare the sauce: Place the garlic in a food processor with the S blade inserted. Mince. Add the peppers. Purée.

3. Pour the purée into a bowl. Add the tofu and mash. Stir in the capers and watercress.

4. Drain the orzo, pour it into the bowl, and toss until all of the ingredients are well mixed.

> **PLANT ESTROGEN ESTIMATE: 1 PORTION PER SERVING**

≋ PASTA WITH CREAMY SAUCES

Here's another way to saturate pasta with plant estrogens—make a creamy sauce. Pull out the food processor. Purée tofu. Infuse it with irresistible flavors. You've got a dieter's dream—the goodness of cream without the saturated fat–filled calories. Instead, you've made a high-protein dish rich with plant estrogens.

But here's a warning: Don't toss creamy tofu sauces with hot pasta. I've done it—tossed a perfectly light, creamy sauce into perfectly al dente pasta. The dish was a lovely mix of sauce and pasta. However, in 10 minutes, the sauce was absorbed directly into each piece of pasta: The pasta was too soft and the sauce was too thick. But the deterioration of a perfect pasta dish can easily be avoided. Just remember to rinse the pasta and serve the sauce on the side.

SMOKED MACKEREL–DIJON SAUCE WITH FETTUCCINE

Work and Cooking Time: *under 15 minutes*
Equipment: *electric food processor*
Yield: *Makes 4 servings*

A light, creamy sauce with a smoked flavor. This dish feels elegantly Italian.

8 ounces fettuccine
2 garlic cloves, quartered
½ cup soy milk
½ cake (9½ ounces) silken tofu

1 tablespoon Dijon mustard
1 teaspoon tamari
4 ounces smoked mackerel fillet

1. Bring 2 quarts of water to a boil. Add the fettuccine and cook for 10 to 12 minutes (or according to package directions).

2. While the pasta cooks, prepare the sauce: Place the garlic in a food processor with the S blade inserted. Mince. Add the soy milk, tofu, mustard, and tamari. Process until smooth. Taste. If needed, add more mustard and tamari. Pour into a saucepan. Remove the skin from the mackerel fillet. Cut the fish into ½-inch pieces. Stir them into the sauce. Heat over medium heat without boiling.

3. Drain and rinse the pasta. Serve the sauce and pasta in separate serving bowls. Pour the sauce over individual servings of pasta at the table.

PLANT ESTROGEN ESTIMATE: ⅔ PORTION PER SERVING

LINGUINE TOSSED WITH CILANTRO
AND ROASTED GARLIC

Work and Cooking Time: *under 15 minutes*
Equipment: *electric food processor*
Yield: *Makes 4 servings*

This sauce has a surprisingly delicate flavor.

8 ounces linguine

2 garlic cloves, quartered

½ cake (9½ ounces) silken tofu

½ cup soy milk

1 tablespoon lime juice

½ cup fresh cilantro

½ cup bottled roasted garlic

Salt

1. Bring 2 quarts of water to a boil. Add the linguine and cook for about 10 minutes (or according to package directions).

2. While the pasta cooks, prepare the sauce: Place the garlic in a food processor with the S blade inserted. Mince. Add the tofu, soy milk, lime juice, and cilantro. Measure ¼ cup of the roasted garlic into the food processor. Process until smooth. Pour into a serving bowl. Chop the remaining garlic coarsely. Stir in. Salt to taste.

3. Drain and rinse the pasta. Serve the sauce and pasta in separate serving bowls. Pour the sauce over individual servings of pasta at the table.

PLANT ESTROGEN ESTIMATE: ⅔ PORTION PER SERVING

BOW TIES, BABY PEAS, AND SALMON

Work and Cooking Time: *under 20 minutes*
Equipment: *electric food processor*
Yield: *Makes 4 servings*

Fun pasta in pink and green—this dish packs a whole meal's worth of nutrition along with its natural estrogens. With peas for a vegetable, tofu and salmon for protein, and pasta for carbohydrate, it's a one-dish marvel.

8 ounces bow-tie pasta
4 garlic cloves, quartered
½ cake (9½ ounces) silken tofu
¾ cup soy milk
2 tablespoons snipped fresh dill

⅔ cup fresh or frozen peas
8 ounces skinless salmon, sliced into 1×3-inch
  strips
2 teaspoons Dijon mustard
Salt and pepper

1. Bring 3 quarts of water to a boil. Add the pasta and cook for about 10 minutes (or according to package directions).

2. While the pasta cooks, prepare the sauce: Place the garlic in a food processor with the S blade inserted. Mince. Add the tofu. Process until smooth.

3. Turn the tofu mixture into a saucepan. Add the soy milk, dill, peas, and salmon. Cook over medium heat, without boiling, until the peas and salmon are cooked. Remove from the heat. Stir in the mustard. Add salt and pepper to taste.

4. Drain and rinse the pasta. Serve the sauce and pasta in separate serving bowls. Pour the sauce over individual servings of pasta at the table.

PLANT ESTROGEN ESTIMATE: ¾ PORTION PER SERVING

SMOKED TOMATO CREME SAUCE
OVER ANGEL HAIR PASTA

Work and Cooking Time: *under 15 minutes*
Equipment: *electric food processor*
Yield: *Makes 4 servings*

Where does the smoked flavor come from? Don't tell: It's the bacin bits. These little pieces of phony meat may be an affront to both gourmet and health-food sensibilities, but it's mere prejudice. Perfectly natural bacin bits can be bought in the most discerning of health food stores! Colored with beets, they add a pink tinge to this creamy sauce.

3 garlic cloves, quartered
15-ounce can diced tomatoes in juice
½ cake (8 ounces) soft tofu
1 tablespoon bacin bits

1 teaspoon dried basil or 1 tablespoon fresh basil
8 ounces angel hair pasta

1. Place the garlic in a food processor with the S blade inserted. Mince. Add the tomatoes, tofu, bacin bits, and basil. Process until creamy. Turn into a saucepan and cook over low heat, being careful not to simmer; this mixture will curdle easily.

2. Bring 2 quarts of water to a boil. Add the pasta and cook for about 3 minutes (or according to package directions). Be careful not to overcook.

3. Remove the sauce from the heat.

4. Drain and rinse the pasta. Serve the sauce and pasta in separate serving bowls. Pour the sauce over individual servings of pasta at the table.

PLANT ESTROGEN ESTIMATE: ½ PORTION PER SERVING

PENNE AND SAUSAGE IN CREAMY TOMATO SAUCE

Work and Cooking Time: *under 20 minutes*
Equipment: *electric food processor*
Yield: *Makes 4 servings*

A hearty dish that can serve as a main course rich in vitamins, protein, and natural estrogens.

Olive-oil spray	⅛ teaspoon black pepper
1 onion, chopped	1 teaspoon bacin bits
2 garlic cloves, chopped	8 ounces penne
12 soy sausages, sliced	½ cake (8 ounces) soft tofu
15-ounce can diced tomatoes in juice	¼ cup soy milk

1. Spray a heavy frying pan with olive oil. Place over medium-high heat. Add the onion, garlic, and sausage. Cook until the onion is lightly browned. Add the tomatoes, pepper, and bacin bits. Simmer.

2. Bring 3 quarts of water to a boil. Add the penne and cook for about 10 minutes (or according to package directions).

3. Place the tofu and soy milk in a food processor with the S blade inserted. Process for 3 minutes, until smooth and silky.

4. Remove the tomato and sausage sauce from the heat. Whisk in the tofu and soy milk.

5. Drain and rinse the pasta. Serve the sauce and pasta in separate serving bowls. Pour the sauce over individual servings of pasta at the table.

PLANT ESTROGEN ESTIMATE: 1¼ PORTIONS PER SERVING

NOODLES WITH CREAMY SESAME SAUCE

Work and Cooking Time: *under 15 minutes*
Equipment: *electric food processor*
Yield: *Makes 4 servings*

Don't expect this to be the usual Chinese sesame-noodle dish. The sauce is creamier.

3 garlic cloves, quartered

1 tablespoon tahini

1 tablespoon peanut butter

1 tablespoon tamari

½ cup unsweetened soy milk

1 cake (18 ounces) silken tofu

12 ounces fresh Chinese noodles

2 tablespoons lime juice

2 tablespoons unhulled sesame seeds

2 tablespoons chopped fresh cilantro

1. Place the garlic in a food processor with the S blade inserted. Mince. Add the tahini, peanut butter, tamari, soy milk, and tofu and process until smooth. Heat in a heavy-bottomed saucepan over medium heat without boiling.

2. While the sauce is heating, bring 2 quarts of water to a boil. Add the noodles and cook for 3 to 5 minutes.

3. Pour the sauce into a serving bowl; stir in the lime juice. Sprinkle the sesame seeds and cilantro over the sauce. Drain and rinse the noodles. Serve the sauce and noodles separately, ladling sauce over the noodles at the table.

PLANT ESTROGEN ESTIMATE: 1 PORTION PER SERVING

MUSHROOM STROGANOFF

Work and Cooking Time: *under 20 minutes*
Equipment: *electric food processor*
Yield: *Makes 4 servings*

No cream here! This stroganoff dish brings you a wealth of plant estrogens in a sauce that feels fattening but isn't.

If you're so inclined, you can make this mushroom dish into a more traditional meat dish. Just sauté cubes of beef or chicken in a frying pan and add to the stroganoff before spooning it over the noodles.

12 ounces broad noodles	2 teaspoons ground cumin
8 garlic cloves, pressed	1 cake (19 ounces) silken tofu
4 cups sliced mushrooms	½ cup soy milk
2 tablespoons tamari	1 tablespoon tahini

1. Bring 4 quarts of water to a boil. Add the noodles and cook for about 7 minutes (or according to package directions).

2. While the noodles cook, make the sauce: Heat a heavy-bottomed frying pan over medium-high heat. Add ¼ cup of water. Add the garlic and mushrooms. Cover.

3. Place all of the remaining ingredients in a food processor with the S blade inserted. Process until the mixture is smooth and silky. Taste. If needed, add more tamari and cumin.

4. When the mushrooms have darkened, pour the sauce from the processor into the frying pan. Heat without boiling.

5. As soon as the noodles are cooked al dente, drain, rinse, and pour onto a serving platter.

6. Serve the sauce and the noodles in separate serving bowls. Pour the sauce over individual servings of noodles at the table.

PLANT ESTROGEN ESTIMATE: 1 PORTION PER SERVING

THAI-STYLE NOODLES

Work and Cooking Time: *under 20 minutes*
Equipment: *electric blender*
Yield: *Makes 4 servings*

An Americanized version of *pad Thai,* this dish combines many traditional Thai ingredients with readily available foods. With sprouts, noodles, and tofu, it makes a balanced one-dish meal.

8 ounces linguine	2 tablespoons peanut butter
½ cup soy nuts	⅓ cup soy milk
2 garlic cloves, quartered	½ cake (8 ounces) soft tofu, mashed
2 tablespoons lime juice	2 cups mung bean sprouts
1 tablespoon tamari	3 tablespoons chopped fresh cilantro

1. Bring 2 quarts of water to a boil. Add the linguine and cook for about 10 minutes (or according to package directions).

2. Place the soy nuts in a food processor with the S blade inserted. Process until the nuts are coarsely chopped. Pour into a bowl and set aside.

3. Place the garlic in the food processor. Mince. Add the lime juice, tamari, peanut butter, and soy milk. Process until smooth. Set aside.

4. Drain and rinse the pasta. Place in a bowl. Add the mashed tofu and sprouts. Mix together. Add the peanut butter–lime sauce. Toss. Add the cilantro and toss.

PLANT ESTROGEN ESTIMATE: 1 PORTION PER SERVING

RICE DISHES

Italian risotto inspired these rice-and-flaxseed dishes. Real risotto requires time and culinary commitment. Broth is stirred into cooking rice ½ cup at a time. In the end, the constant stirring produces an unusual rice dish—a combination of soft and firm grains encased in a creamy sauce. With flaxseed and tofu, you get a shortcut to risotto; you get the feel of risotto without a half hour of stirring. Together, the two estrogenic ingredients surround the rice with a tasty sauce.

SPINACH-AND-SUN-DRIED TOMATO RISOTTO

Work Time: *under 10 minutes*
Cooking Time: *1 hour*
Equipment: *electric food processor*
Yield: *Makes 4 servings*

A wonderful combination of unusual tastes in a very easy dish.

¾ cup short-grain brown rice

10 ounces fresh or frozen spinach, chopped

⅓ cup chopped sun-dried tomatoes

3 garlic cloves, minced

2 tablespoons brown miso

½ cake (9½ ounces) silken tofu

¼ cup flaxseed

1. Bring 2 cups of water to a boil in a heavy-bottomed pot. Add the rice. Reduce the heat to a simmer. Cover and cook for 50 minutes.

2. Stir in the spinach, sun-dried tomatoes, garlic, and miso and cook uncovered for 10 minutes. Purée the tofu in a food processor with the S blade inserted and stir it into the rice. Add the flaxseed. Stir until thoroughly combined and creamy. Serve.

PLANT ESTROGEN ESTIMATE: 1½ PORTIONS PER SERVING

SESAME RISOTTO

Work Time: *10 minutes*
Cooking Time: *55 minutes*
Equipment: *electric food processor*
Yield: *Makes 4 servings*

Crunchy and creamy—a sesame delight.

⅔ cup short-grain brown rice
3 garlic cloves, quartered
1 tablespoon brown miso
1 tablespoon tahini

½ cake (9½ ounces) silken tofu
1 tablespoon sesame seeds
¼ cup flaxseed

1. Bring 1½ cups of water to a boil in a heavy-bottomed pot. Add the rice. Reduce the heat to a simmer. Cover and cook for 50 minutes.

2. Place the garlic in a food processor with the S blade inserted. Mince. Add the miso, tahini, and tofu. Process until smooth. Pour into the rice. Add the sesame seeds and flaxseed. Stir. Cook uncovered for 5 minutes without boiling. Serve.

PLANT ESTROGEN ESTIMATE: 1½ PORTIONS PER SERVING

MUSHROOM RISOTTO

Work Time: *10 minutes*
Cooking Time: *55 minutes*
Equipment: *electric food processor*
Yield: *Makes 4 servings*

Creamy, crunchy rice with a delicious mushroom flavor.

⅔ cup short-grain brown rice
Spray oil
1 onion, chopped
3 garlic cloves, sliced
10 ounces mushrooms, sliced

2 tablespoons brown miso
1 teaspoon ground cumin
½ cake (9½ ounces) silken tofu
¼ cup flaxseed

1. Bring 1½ cups of water to a boil in a heavy-bottomed pot. Add the rice. Reduce the heat to a simmer. Cover and cook for 50 minutes.

2. Spray a heavy frying pan with oil. Heat over medium-high heat. Sauté the onion, garlic, and mushrooms until browned. Reduce the heat to low. Add the cooked rice; stir.

3. Place the miso, cumin, and tofu in a food processor with the S blade inserted. Purée. Add to the rice-and-mushroom mixture. Stir. Add the flaxseed. Stir. Cook uncovered for 5 minutes without boiling.

PLANT ESTROGEN ESTIMATE: 1½ PORTIONS PER SERVING

LEMON-ASPARAGUS RISOTTO

Work Time: *10 minutes*
Cooking Time: *55 minutes*
Equipment: *electric food processor*
Yield: *Makes 4 servings*

A springtime special, and a great showcase for fresh asparagus.

⅔ cup short-grain brown rice
4 garlic cloves, quartered
2 tablespoons brown miso
2 tablespoons lemon juice
2 tablespoons Dijon mustard

2 teaspoons grated lemon rind
½ cake (9½ ounces) silken tofu
¾ cup chopped asparagus
¼ cup flaxseed

1. Bring 1½ cups of water to a boil in a heavy-bottomed pot. Add the rice. Reduce the heat to a simmer. Cover and cook for 50 minutes.

2. Place the garlic in a food processor with the S blade inserted. Mince. Add the miso, lemon juice, mustard, lemon rind, and tofu. Process until smooth.

3. Stir the mixture into the cooked rice. Reduce the heat to low. Stir in the asparagus and flaxseed. Cook uncovered, stirring constantly, until the asparagus is bright green and crisp. Serve.

PLANT ESTROGEN ESTIMATE: 1¼ PORTIONS PER SERVING

CURRIED RICE WITH PEAS

Work Time: *under 10 minutes*
Cooking Time: *50 minutes*
Equipment: *electric food processor*
Yield: *Makes 4 servings*

This dish is a cross-cultural experience: It has a texture like Italian risotto and tastes like Indian pilaf.

¾ cup brown rice
Canola-oil spray
1 onion, chopped
3 garlic cloves, sliced
⅔ cup fresh or frozen peas
6 ⅛×1-inch slices fresh ginger

1 teaspoon curry powder
½ teaspoon ground coriander
½ teaspoon turmeric
¼ cup flaxseed
½ cake (9½ ounces) silken tofu
2 tablespoons yellow miso

1. Bring 1½ cups of water to a boil in a heavy-bottomed pot. Add the rice. Reduce the heat to a simmer. Cover and cook for 45 minutes or until tender.

2. Spray a heavy-bottomed frying pan with oil. Sauté the onion and garlic until browned. Add the peas, ginger, curry powder, coriander, and turmeric. Stir in the cooked rice and the flaxseed.

3. Purée the tofu and miso in a food processor with the S blade inserted. Stir into the rice mixture. Heat. Serve.

PLANT ESTROGEN ESTIMATE: 1½ PORTIONS PER SERVING

Ten

Main Dishes

My advice: Don't depend entirely on main dishes to eat estrogen daily. You and your family will get bored and discouraged. Eat an estrogenic main dish only when you feel like it. When you want a quiche, a curry, a casserole, a loaf, a Chinese stir-fry, or a fish dish, turn to the recipes in this chapter. If you never get the urge for a main dish made with soy or flaxseed, don't worry. You can get your daily dose of plant estrogen munching breakfast foods, snacks, and desserts.

〰 CURRIES

If you're already fighting off hot flashes, highly spiced food is not an ally. A dish that can make your mouth burn and your face sweat may make your entire body heat up. You may want to keep these curries on the mild side.

SPINACH CURRY

Work and Cooking Time: *10 minutes*
Equipment: *electric food processor*
Yield: *Makes 4 servings*

Light green and creamy, with a strong ginger taste.

3 garlic cloves, quartered
4 ⅛×1-inch slices fresh ginger
1 cake (16 ounces) soft tofu
2 tablespoons soy milk

1 tablespoon frozen apple juice concentrate
Salt
16 ounces fresh or frozen spinach, chopped

1. Place the garlic and ginger in a food processor with the S blade inserted. Mince. Add the tofu, soy milk, and apple juice concentrate. Process until smooth. Salt to taste.
2. Pour the mixture into a heavy frying pan. Add the spinach. Heat, without boiling, stirring occasionally. Serve.

PLANT ESTROGEN ESTIMATE: **1** PORTION PER SERVING

YELLOW CAULIFLOWER CURRY

Work and Cooking Time: *under 20 minutes*
Equipment: *electric food processor*
Yield: *Makes 4 servings*

A creamy, bright-yellow sauce turns steamed cauliflower into an Indian delicacy.

3 cups cauliflower florets

4 garlic cloves, quartered

4 ⅛×1-inch slices fresh ginger

1 teaspoon turmeric

1 teaspoon curry powder

2 teaspoons frozen apple juice concentrate

¼ cup soy milk

1 cake (16 ounces) soft tofu

3 tablespoons chopped fresh cilantro

1. Steam the cauliflower over 2 cups of water until just tender.

2. While the cauliflower steams, prepare the curry sauce: Place the garlic in a food processor with the S blade inserted. Mince. Add the ginger. Mince. Add the turmeric, curry powder, apple juice concentrate, soy milk, and tofu. Process for 4 minutes, until creamy.

3. Pour the sauce into a heavy-bottomed frying pan. Add the steamed cauliflower and cook over medium heat without boiling, stirring occasionally. Remove from the heat. Stir in the cilantro. Serve.

PLANT ESTROGEN ESTIMATE: 1 PORTION PER SERVING

VARIATION: Substitute pieces of sautéed chicken breast for the cauliflower.

THAI-STYLE YELLOW CURRY

Work and Cooking Time: *under 25 minutes*
Baking Time: *under 20 minutes*
Equipment: *electric food processor*
Yield: *Makes 4 servings*

Traditional Thai yellow curry is a no-no: Made with coconut milk and deep-fried tofu, it's high in cholesterol and fat. Substitute this heart-saving sauce and oven-roasted tofu and it's transformed—so healthy you could live on it. It has vegetables, fruit, protein, and calcium all in one dish. Plus, it's an exceptional source of plant estrogens.

This recipe uses fresh ginger to make a lovely curry sauce. If you can find Thai curry paste, the dish will taste more Thai-like. Look at the package ingredients. The best curry paste for this dish will have lemongrass and ginger. Often it's used to make coconut soup.

To use Thai curry paste in the recipe, leave out the ginger. Add the paste instead of salting to taste. Stir the curry paste in ½ teaspoon at a time until it tastes perfect. This saucy dish goes well with rice.

1 cake (16 ounces) firm tofu
Canola-oil spray
1 onion, cut into 8 wedges
1 fresh pineapple, peeled, cored, and cut into 1-inch chunks
1 green bell pepper, cut into 1-inch pieces
1 red bell pepper, cut into 1-inch pieces

6 garlic cloves, quartered
6 ⅛×1-inch slices fresh ginger
1 cake (19 ounces) silken tofu
2 tablespoons yellow miso
¾ teaspoon turmeric
½ teaspoon honey

1. Preheat the oven to 500°F.

2. Cut the firm tofu into triangles: First cut the cake in half, making two rectangles. Cut the halves into triangles by cutting them from corner to corner. Slice each triangle twice, making twelve triangles about ½ inch thick. Arrange on a broiler pan. Spray with oil. Turn over and spray again. Place in the oven. Roast until lightly golden on the undersides, 5 to 10 minutes. Turn over. Roast until the bottoms are golden, another 5 to 10 minutes.

3. While the tofu roasts, prepare the vegetables: Spray a frying pan with oil. Heat the pan over high heat. Add the onion and pineapple. When the onion is heated but still crisp, add the green and red pepper. Reduce the heat to medium. Heat the vegetables without overcooking them—they should be hot and crisp.

4. While the vegetables cook, prepare the sauce: Place the garlic in a food processor with the S blade inserted. Mince. Add the ginger. Mince. Add the tofu, miso, turmeric, and honey. Process until smooth and creamy.

5. Pour the sauce over the heated vegetables. Reduce the heat to low. Add the roasted tofu. Heat without boiling, stirring occasionally. Serve while the vegetables are still crisp.

PLANT ESTROGEN ESTIMATE: **2** PORTIONS PER SERVING

What do I mean by "meaty"? I mean "meatlike"—chewy and salty soy in sauces that usually come with artery-clogging meat.

SWEDISH "MEATBALLS"

≋

Work and Cooking Time: *under 30 minutes*
Equipment: *electric food processor*
Yield: *Makes 4 servings*

I'm of Scandinavian ancestry, and this dish reminds me of my childhood. This variation, however, is a cholesterol-free, health-protecting main course with a double dose of plant estrogens in every serving.

For "meatballs," use a soy ground "beef," found in the refrigerator or freezer section of your health food store. Lightlife, the makers of Smart Dogs, distributes a good-tasting fat-free version.

4 new potatoes, diced

Canola-oil spray

14 ounces soy ground "beef," formed into tablespoon-size balls

4 garlic cloves, quartered

1 cake (19 ounces) silken tofu

⅓ cup plus 2 tablespoons soy milk

2 teaspoons ground cumin

½ teaspoon ground coriander

2 tablespoons tamari

1. Place the potatoes in 1 quart of boiling water. Cook, covered, over medium-high heat.

2. Spray a large frying pan with oil. Heat over medium-high heat. Add the "meatballs" and brown, turning occasionally.

3. Place the garlic in a food processor with the S blade inserted. Mince. Add the tofu, ⅓ cup soy milk, cumin, coriander, and tamari. Process until smooth and creamy. Pour the mixture into the frying pan with the browned "meatballs." Reduce the heat to medium. Cook without boiling, stirring occasionally.

4. When the potatoes are soft, drain and place in a mixing bowl. Add the 2 table-spoons of soy milk. Mash with an electric mixer or potato masher. Serve the "meatballs" and gravy spooned over the potatoes.

PLANT ESTROGEN ESTIMATE: **2** PORTIONS PER SERVING

CHILI WITH BEANS

Work and Cooking Time: *15 minutes*
Yield: *Makes 4 servings*

TVP (texturized vegetable protein) makes great chili. You really might mistake it for ground beef, but there's no fat.

Canola-oil spray
1 onion, chopped
3 garlic cloves, minced
3 tablespoons brown miso
2 15-ounce cans tomato sauce
1 cup dry TVP (texturized vegetable protein)

16-ounce can pinto beans
¼ teaspoon chili powder
½ teaspoon ground cumin
1 teaspoon dried oregano

1. Spray a large frying pan with oil. Heat. Sauté the onion and garlic until browned.
2. Stir in the miso. Add the remaining ingredients. Cook over medium-high heat until the texturized vegetable protein has a hamburger-like texture and the flavors are combined. Serve.

PLANT ESTROGEN ESTIMATE: **1** PORTION PER SERVING

NOUVEAU CHILI

⧟

Work and Cooking Time: *20 minutes*
Yield: *Makes 4 servings*

Chili with a modern twist.

Canola-oil spray
1 onion, chopped
3 garlic cloves, sliced
2 tablespoons brown miso
2 15-ounce cans tomato sauce
½ cup minced sun-dried tomatoes

1 teaspoon ground cumin
1 teaspoon chili powder
1 teaspoon dried oregano
1 cup dry TVP (textured vegetable protein)
2 tablespoons chopped fresh cilantro

1. Spray a large frying pan with oil. Heat. Sauté the onion and garlic until browned.
2. Stir in the miso. Add the remaining ingredients and ½ cup of water. Cook over medium-high heat until the texturized vegetable protein has a hamburger-like texture and the flavors are combined. Serve.

PLANT ESTROGEN ESTIMATE: **1** PORTION PER SERVING

POTATO-AND-PEPPER STEW

⧟

Work and Cooking Time: *under 25 minutes*
Yield: *Makes 4 servings*

For me, this is nostalgia food; I loved the full-fat version when I was a little girl.

3 new potatoes, cut in ½-inch cubes
Spray oil
2 onions, chopped
4 garlic cloves, sliced
3 tablespoons brown miso

1 teaspoon ground cumin
¼ teaspoon black pepper
3 cups unsweetened soy milk
1 cup dry TVP (texturized vegetable protein)
2 green bell peppers, diced

1. Place the potatoes in a pot. Cover with water. Bring to a boil. Cook until soft.

2. Spray a heavy-bottomed frying pan with oil. Heat over medium-high heat. Sauté the onion and garlic until browned. Add the miso, cumin, and black pepper. Stir until the miso is dissolved. Add the soy milk and TVP. Reduce the heat. Add the potato and green pepper. Cook until the TVP is chewy. Serve.

PLANT ESTROGEN ESTIMATE: 1 PORTION PER SERVING

NUTTY CHILI

Work and Cooking Time: *under 20 minutes*
Equipment: *electric food processor*
Yield: *Makes 4 servings*

Canola-oil spray

2 onions, chopped

5 garlic cloves, sliced

2 tablespoons brown miso

2 tablespoons peanut butter

1 teaspoon chili powder

1 teaspoon ground cumin

2 cups unsweetened soy milk

¾ cup dry TVP (texturized vegetable protein)

½ cup tomato sauce

½ cup soy nuts

⅓ cup chopped fresh cilantro

1. Spray a heavy-bottomed frying pan with oil. Heat over medium-high heat. Sauté the onion and garlic until lightly browned. Reduce the heat to low. Stir in the miso and peanut butter. Add the chili powder, cumin, soy milk, and TVP. Cook for 10 minutes, until the TVP is chewy. Stir in the tomato sauce. Cook without boiling until heated.

2. Place the soy nuts in a food processor with the S blade inserted. Pulse to chop. Sprinkle over the chili. Sprinkle cilantro over the chili. Serve.

PLANT ESTROGEN ESTIMATE: 1½ PORTIONS PER SERVING

SHIITAKE MUSHROOM RING WITH GRAVY

Work and Cooking Time: *under 15 minutes*
Waiting Time: *2 hours*
Baking Time: *1¼ hours*
Equipment: *electric food processor*
Yield: *Makes 8 servings*

The chewy, meaty texture doesn't come from soy. The taste is actually a bit more like oyster than meat. It comes from massive amounts of shiitake mushrooms. If you have to buy them in a gourmet store, this dish will cost a fortune. If you buy them in a Chinese market, however, they won't break the budget.

Ring

4 cups dried shiitake mushrooms

4 garlic cloves, quartered

2 cakes (32 ounces) firm tofu

3 tablespoons brown miso

Gravy

5 garlic cloves, quartered

2 teaspoons tahini

1 cake (19 ounces) silken tofu

2 tablespoons tamari

1. Place the mushrooms in a bowl. Cover with warm water. Allow to soak for 2 hours, until the mushrooms are rehydrated. Drain the mushrooms, but reserve the soaking water.

2. Preheat the oven to 400°F.

3. To make the ring, place the garlic in a food processor with the S blade inserted. Mince. Add about half the mushrooms, 1 cake firm tofu, ¼ cup of the reserved soaking water, and 1½ tablespoons of miso. Purée. Turn into a large mixing bowl. Purée the remaining mushrooms, tofu, and miso and add to the bowl. Combine. Pour the mixture into an 8-inch nonstick or oiled ring mold. Bake for 1 hour and 15 minutes, until the ring is firm.

4. While the ring bakes, prepare the gravy: Place the garlic in a food processor with the S blade inserted. Mince. Add the remaining gravy ingredients plus ½ cup of the reserved soaking water. Process until smooth. Pour into a saucepan and heat over medium-low heat.

5. Unmold the ring. Serve with gravy on the side.

PLANT ESTROGEN ESTIMATE: 1½ PORTIONS PER SERVING

SWEET-AND-SOUR BALLS

Work and Cooking Time: *15 minutes*
Baking Time: *15 minutes*
Yield: *Makes 4 servings*

A real treat—light and crispy balls in a sweet-and-sour sauce—that gives you a double portion of plant estrogens in every serving. Freezing firm tofu and thawing it transforms its smooth feel into a meatlike texture.

Sweet-and-Sour Balls
2 tablespoons peanut butter
2 tablespoons tamari
6 garlic cloves, pressed
2 tablespoons dried cilantro
½ cup finely chopped water chestnuts
½ cup finely chopped scallions
2 cakes (32 ounces) frozen firm tofu, thawed
Canola-oil spray

Sweet-and-Sour Sauce
4 garlic cloves, pressed
1 cup frozen apple juice concentrate
2 tablespoons cornstarch
2 tablespoons apple cider vinegar
1½ tablespoons tamari

1. Preheat the oven to 500°F.

2. To make the balls, cream the peanut butter and tamari in a mixing bowl. Add the garlic, cilantro, water chestnuts, and scallions. Place the tofu between two plates. Press down on the top plate and pour off any water. Crumble the tofu into the bowl. Mash the ingredients until they are thoroughly combined into a meatball-like mixture. Form into balls. Spray each ball lightly with oil. Place on a cookie sheet. Bake for 15 minutes, until the balls are lightly crusty.

3. While the sweet-and-sour balls cook, prepare the sauce: Place the garlic and apple juice concentrate in a heavy-bottomed saucepan. Place over medium-high heat. Dissolve the cornstarch in the vinegar and tamari. When the apple juice concentrate begins to boil, whisk in the dissolved cornstarch mixture. Stir continually until the sauce is thickened and translucent. Remove from the heat. Pour the sauce over the balls and coat them evenly just before serving.

> **PLANT ESTROGEN ESTIMATE: 2 PORTIONS PER SERVING**

There's no need to limit your traditional recipes to the recipes in this cookbook. Check out Chinese cookbooks. You'll find a wealth of estrogenic main dishes.

FAMILY-STYLE TOFU

≋

Work and Cooking Time: *under 25 minutes*
Baking Time: *under 20 minutes*
Yield: *Makes 4 servings*

I was pregnant when I discovered this traditional Chinese dish. It became an obsession—a true craving. Every day for a month, I went to the same restaurant and ordered Family-style Tofu. I most loved the texture of the deep-fried tofu, a delicacy I knew I had to forsake to take better care of myself. Imagine my excitement when I concocted a healthier alternative—roasted tofu. Now, I can make my favorite Chinese dish and enjoy the naturally estrogenic results.

1½ cakes (24 ounces) firm tofu	6 garlic cloves, chopped
Canola-oil spray	8 ⅛×1-inch slices fresh ginger
2 onions, sliced	2 tablespoons tamari
2 carrots, sliced	1 tablespoon cornstarch

1. Preheat the oven to 500°F.

2. Cut the tofu into triangles: First cut the whole cake in half, making two rectangles. Cut the three halves (1½ cakes) into triangles by cutting them from corner to corner. Slice each triangle twice, making eighteen triangles about ½ inch thick. Arrange on a broiler pan. Spray with oil. Turn over and spray again. Place in the oven. Roast until lightly golden on the undersides, 5 to 10 minutes. Turn over. Roast until the bottoms are golden, another 5 to 10 minutes.

3. While the tofu roasts, prepare the vegetables and sauce: Spray a frying pan with oil and heat over medium-high heat. Add the onion, carrot, garlic, and ginger. Sauté until

the onion is browned and the carrot can be easily pierced with a fork. Increase the heat to high. Add the tamari and ¾ cup of water. In a small bowl, dissolve the cornstarch in 2 tablespoons of water. Stir in. Continue stirring until the sauce thickens. Remove from the heat. Add the roasted tofu. Mix until the tofu is thoroughly coated.

PLANT ESTROGEN ESTIMATE: 1½ PORTIONS PER SERVING

TOFU WITH SHIITAKE MUSHROOMS AND GREENS

Work and Cooking Time: *under 20 minutes*
Waiting time: *2 hours*
Yield: *Makes 4 servings*

In this dish, you'll find a nutritional treasure chest: natural estrogen, protein, and calcium.

1 cup dried shiitake mushrooms	1 cake (16 ounces) soft tofu, cut into 2-inch
3 cloves garlic, minced	squares (½ inch thick)
1 tablespoon grated fresh ginger	3 cups (4 ounces) young, tender watercress
2 tablespoons tamari	3 cups (4 ounces) arugula
1 tablespoon cornstarch	3 cups pea greens or spinach

1. Place the mushrooms in a bowl. Cover with warm water. Allow to soak for 2 hours, until the mushrooms are rehydrated. Squeeze the water out of the mushrooms and set aside. Reserve the soaking water.

2. Measure 1 cup of the soaking water into a frying pan. Add the mushrooms, garlic, and ginger. Cook over medium-high heat. Dissolve the tamari and cornstarch in 2 tablespoons water. When the liquid begins to simmer, stir in the dissolved tamari and cornstarch. Stir while the sauce thickens. Add the tofu. Reduce the heat to low.

3. Steam the greens in a steamer over 2 cups of water for 5 minutes or until tender. Add the steamed greens to the tofu in brown sauce. Remove from the heat and serve.

PLANT ESTROGEN ESTIMATE: 1 PORTION PER SERVING

Tofu does egg well. Whether it's quiche, custard, or crêpes, tofu replicates these conventional egg dishes with ease. The density of the tofu makes an enormous difference. Be sure to use extra-firm tofu for quiche, firm for crêpes, and silken for custard.

CRUSTLESS MUSHROOM QUICHE

🟰

Work and Cooking Time: *under 15 minutes*
Baking Time: *50 minutes*
Equipment: *electric food processor*
Yield: *Makes 6 servings*

When this quiche is fully cooked, the top resembles parched earth—not very attractive. To make the quiche more presentable, treat it like a loaf: Take it out of the oven, cover it with a dinner plate, turn it over, and remove the pie plate.

Canola-oil spray
1 onion, chopped
3 cups sliced fresh mushrooms
5 garlic cloves, quartered
4 ⅛×1-inch slices fresh ginger

1½ cakes (24 ounces) extra-firm tofu
¼ teaspoon turmeric
2 teaspoons ground cumin
2 tablespoons tamari

1. Preheat the oven to 350°F.
2. Spray a heavy frying pan with canola oil. Sauté the onion and mushrooms until browned.
3. While the vegetables sauté, prepare the quiche mixture: Place the garlic in a food processor with the S blade inserted. Mince. Add the ginger. Mince. Break the tofu into small pieces and place in the food processor. Add the remaining ingredients. Process for at least 3 minutes, until smooth. Taste. If needed, add more cumin.

4. Turn the mixture into a bowl. Add the sautéed onion and mushrooms. Mix until thoroughly distributed. Turn into a 9-inch nonstick or oiled pie plate. Bake for 50 minutes, until set. Unmold. Allow to cool for 5 minutes before serving.

PLANT ESTROGEN ESTIMATE: 1 PORTION PER SERVING

MACKEREL-AND-ONION QUICHE

Work Time: *under 15 minutes*
Baking Time: *50 minutes*
Equipment: *electric food processor*
Yield: *Makes 6 servings*

Smoked mackerel is a reasonably priced way to get the flavor of smoked fish. But if you prefer the taste and color of smoked salmon, you can easily substitute lox for mackerel.

5 garlic cloves, quartered
1½ cakes (24 ounces) extra-firm tofu
3 tablespoons Dijon mustard

¼ teaspoon turmeric
8 ounces smoked mackerel, cut into bits
1 onion, chopped

1. Preheat the oven to 350°F.
2. Place the garlic in a food processor with the S blade inserted. Mince. Break the tofu into small pieces and place in the food processor Add the mustard and turmeric. Process for at least 3 minutes, until smooth. Taste. If needed, add more mustard.
3. Turn the mixture into a bowl. Add the smoked fish and onion. Mix until thoroughly distributed. Turn into a 9-inch nonstick or oiled pie plate. Bake for 50 minutes, until set. Allow to cool for 5 minutes before serving.

PLANT ESTROGEN ESTIMATE: 1 PORTION PER SERVING

SPINACH QUICHE

≋

Work Time: *under 15 minutes*
Baking Time: *1 hour*
Equipment: *electric food processor*
Yield: *Makes 6 servings*

This colorful quiche has a light nutmeg flavor.

4 garlic cloves, quartered
1½ cakes (24 ounces) extra-firm tofu
½ teaspoon turmeric
½ teaspoon ground nutmeg
3 tablespoons Dijon mustard

1 onion, chopped
20 ounces fresh spinach, steamed and chopped, or frozen chopped spinach, thawed

1. Preheat the oven to 350°F.

2. Place the garlic in a food processor with the S blade inserted. Mince. Break the tofu into small pieces and place in the food processor. Add the turmeric, nutmeg, and mustard. Process for 3 minutes, until smooth.

3. Turn into a medium-size mixing bowl. Add the onion. Squeeze all the water out of the spinach. Add. Mix until thoroughly combined. Turn into a 9-inch nonstick or oiled pie plate. Bake for 1 hour, until set. Unmold onto a dinner plate. Allow to cool for 5 minutes before serving.

PLANT ESTROGEN ESTIMATE: 1 PORTION PER SERVING

FOO YONG

Work Time: *under 10 minutes*
Baking Time: *40 minutes*
Equipment: *electric food processor*
Yield: *Makes 2 servings*

This variation of a traditional Chinese dish has a strong taste of ginger.

3 garlic cloves, quartered
5 ⅛×1-inch slices fresh ginger
1 cake (16 ounces) extra-firm tofu
3 tablespoons Dijon mustard

¼ teaspoon turmeric
1 onion, chopped
2 cups mung bean sprouts

1. Preheat the oven to 350°F.

2. Place the garlic in a food processor with the S blade inserted. Mince. Add the ginger. Mince. Break the tofu into small pieces and place in the food processor. Add the mustard and turmeric. Process for 3 minutes, until smooth.

3. Turn into a bowl. Mix in the onion and sprouts until thoroughly combined.

4. Turn into an 11-inch oiled or nonstick frying pan. Spread evenly. Bake for 40 minutes, until set. Cool for 5 minutes before serving.

PLANT ESTROGEN ESTIMATE: **2** PORTIONS PER SERVING

CURRIED MUSHROOM CUSTARD

Work Time: *under 15 minutes*
Baking Time: *1 hour*
Equipment: *electric food processor*
Yield: *Makes 4 servings*

Made like dessert custards, these creamy little dinner concoctions melt in your mouth.

Canola-oil spray	6 ⅛×1-inch slices fresh ginger
1 onion, chopped	1 tablespoon yellow miso
2½ cups sliced mushrooms	2 teaspoons curry powder
3 garlic cloves, quartered	1 cake (19 ounces) silken tofu

1. Preheat the oven to 250°F.

2. Spray a heavy frying pan with oil. Heat over medium-high heat. Sauté the onion and mushrooms until browned. Remove from the heat. Turn into a mixing bowl.

3. Place the garlic in a food processor with the S blade inserted. Mince. Add the ginger. Mince. Add the miso, curry powder, and tofu. Purée until smooth and creamy. Pour into the mixing bowl with the onion and mushrooms. Stir until well combined.

4. Spoon the mixture into four 8-ounce individual custard cups. Place the filled custard cups in a pan with 1 inch of water. Place the pan in the oven. Bake for 1 hour, until the custard is set. Serve.

PLANT ESTROGEN ESTIMATE: 1 PORTION PER SERVING

BASIC DINNER CRÊPES

Work Time: *under 10 minutes*
Baking Time: *8 to 10 minutes*
Equipment: *electric food processor*
Yield: *Makes 2 servings of 2 crêpes*

Any of your favorite fillings can be folded into these basic dinner crêpes.

1 cake (16 ounces) firm tofu
1 tablespoon tamari

Canola-oil spray
Filling of choice

1. Preheat the oven to 500°F.

2. Place the tofu and tamari in a food processor with the S blade inserted. Process for 2 minutes, until smooth and silky.

3. Spray four 9-inch round cake pans with oil. Spoon the tofu mixture into the center of each, dividing the mixture evenly. Using the back of a soup spoon, carefully spread the tofu mixture, making expanding circles and gradually moving the mixture toward the edge of the pans. Do not allow the mixture to touch the edge of the cake pans. Distribute the batter as evenly as possible, leaving the outer edge of the batter slightly thicker than the middle. This will prevent uneven cooking or spotty burning.

4. Bake for 8 to 10 minutes, until the edges of the crêpes are brown, the batter has a crêpelike texture, and the crêpes can be folded without breaking. Remove from the oven before the edges become crisp.

5. While still in the cake pans, gently fold the crêpes in half and then in quarters. Using a spatula, move the folded crêpes to a serving plate. Unfold. Spoon filling down the center of each crêpe. Fold the crêpe over the filling. Serve.

PLANT ESTROGEN ESTIMATE: **2** PORTIONS PER SERVING

MUSHROOM CRÊPES

Work and Cooking Time: *30 minutes*
Baking Time: *8 to 10 minutes*
Equipment: *electric food processor*
Yield: *Makes 2 servings of 2 crêpes*

Filling
Canola-oil spray
2 garlic cloves, minced
16 ounces fresh mushrooms, chopped
1 teaspoon tamari

Sauce
¼ cake (4¾ ounces) silken tofu
½ cup unsweetened soy milk
1 tablespoon tamari
¼ cup reserved sautéed mushrooms

1 recipe Basic Dinner Crêpes (page 219)

1. To prepare the filling, spray a frying pan with oil. Heat over medium-high heat. Add the garlic and mushrooms. Sauté. Stir in the tamari.

2. To prepare the sauce, place all of the sauce ingredients in a food processor with the S blade inserted. Process until smooth. Pour into a saucepan. Heat over low heat without boiling.

3. Fill the crêpes with mushroom filling and spoon the sauce over them.

PLANT ESTROGEN ESTIMATE: **2¾ PORTIONS PER SERVING**

ASPARAGUS CRÊPES

Work and Cooking Time: *30 minutes*
Baking Time: *8 to 10 minutes*
Equipment: *electric food processor*
Yield: *Makes 2 servings of 2 crêpes*

Crêpes
1 cake (16 ounces) firm tofu
1 tablespoon tamari
½ teaspoon lemon juice
Canola-oil spray

Sauce
2 garlic cloves, quartered
½ cup unsweetened soy milk

½ cake (9½ ounces) silken tofu
1 tablespoon tamari
2 tablespoons lemon juice

Filling
16 ounces asparagus

1. To prepare the crêpes, preheat the oven to 500°F.

2. Place the tofu, tamari, and lemon juice in a food processor with the S blade inserted. Process for 2 minutes, until smooth.

3. Spray four 9-inch round cake pans with oil. Spoon the tofu mixture into the center of each, dividing the mixture evenly. Using the back of a soup spoon, carefully spread the tofu mixture, making expanding circles and gradually moving the mixture toward the edge of the pans. Do not allow the batter to touch the edge of the cake pans. Distribute the batter as evenly as possible, leaving the outer edge of the batter slightly thicker than the middle. This will prevent uneven cooking or spotty burning.

4. Bake for 8 to 10 minutes, until the edges of the crêpes are brown, the batter has a crêpelike texture, and the crêpes can be folded without breaking. Remove the crêpes from the oven before the edges become crisp.

5. While the crêpes bake, prepare the sauce and filling: Place the garlic in a food processor with the S blade inserted. Mince. Add the soy milk and tofu. Purée until smooth. Pour into a saucepan and heat.

6. Steam the asparagus until the color brightens and the spears are crisp.

7. While still in the cake pans, gently fold the crêpes in half and then in quarters. Using a spatula, move the folded crêpes to two serving plates. Unfold. Place a serving of asparagus on each crêpe. Fold the crêpes over the asparagus.

8. Remove the sauce from the heat. Stir in the tamari and lemon juice. Taste. If needed, add more tamari or lemon juice. Spoon the sauce over the filled crêpes. Serve.

PLANT ESTROGEN ESTIMATE: 3¼ PORTIONS PER SERVING

≋ FISH DISHES

Fish is the only flesh food in this cookbook. It's just too good for your heart and your bones not to be included.

BREADED SOLE WITH NUT BUTTER

≋

Work and Cooking Time: *under 25 minutes*
Equipment: *electric food processor and electric coffee grinder*
Yield: *Makes 4 servings*

Avoid deep-fried food! That health message has reached us all. This fish is oven-baked, but the nutty breading provides just enough crispness to be satisfying. The nut butter adds additional natural estrogen.

1 garlic clove, quartered
½ cake (8 ounces) soft tofu
3 tablespoons soy milk
1 teaspoon cashew or almond butter
Salt
1¼ cups soy nuts
4 6-ounce sole fillets
Canola-oil spray

Nut Butter
1 garlic clove, quartered
¼ cake (4 ounces) soft tofu
2 tablespoons high-lignan flax oil
1 tablespoon cashew or almond butter
1½ tablespoons chopped walnuts

1. Preheat the broiler.

2. Place the garlic in a food processor with the S blade inserted. Mince. Add the tofu, soy milk, and cashew butter. Process until smooth. Salt to taste. Pour the batter into a 9-inch pie plate.

3. Grind the soy nuts in an electric coffee grinder ⅓ cup at a time. Pour onto a flat plate.

4. Dip a sole fillet into the tofu batter, coating it thoroughly. Dip it into the ground soy nuts, coating it evenly. Spray with oil on both sides. Place on a broiler pan. Repeat for each fillet.

5. Broil until the tops are lightly browned and crisp. Turn over and broil on the other side.

6. While the fish broils, prepare the nut butter: Place the garlic in a food processor with the S blade inserted. Mince. Add the tofu, oil, and nut butter. Process until smooth and silky. Turn into a small bowl. Stir in the nuts.

7. Serve the fish with nut butter spooned on top.

PLANT ESTROGEN ESTIMATE: **2** PORTIONS PER SERVING

BROILED BLUEFISH WITH
ROASTED RED PEPPER-AND-BASIL SAUCE

Work and Cooking Time: *under 15 minutes*
Equipment: *electric food processor*
Yield: *Makes 4 servings*

The bright red-and-green sauce gives this dish a festive feel.

Spray oil

4 pieces (about 1½ pounds) bluefish

Sauce

3 garlic cloves, quartered

6-ounce jar roasted red peppers, drained

¼ cup fresh basil leaves

½ cake (8 ounces) soft tofu

1 tablespoon lemon juice

Salt

4 slices lime

1. Preheat the broiler.

2. Spray both sides of the bluefish fillets with oil. Place the fillets on a broiler pan, skin side up. Broil for 3 to 5 minutes, until the skin is lightly browned and even bubbly.

3. While the fish broils, prepare the sauce: Place the garlic in a food processor with the S blade inserted. Mince. Add the peppers, basil, tofu, and lemon juice. Process until smooth. Salt to taste.

4. Pour the sauce onto a serving platter. Arrange the broiled fish on top of the sauce. Place one slice of lime on each fillet. Serve.

PLANT ESTROGEN ESTIMATE: ½ PORTION PER SERVING

FLOUNDER WITH GARLIC-DILL SAUCE

Work and Cooking Time: *under 15 minutes*
Equipment: *electric food processor*
Yield: *Makes 4 servings*

If flounder isn't available, this delicate dill sauce makes a delicious companion for sole, tilapia, bass, or any white-fish fillet.

2 garlic cloves, quartered
½ cake (9½ ounces) silken tofu
2 tablespoons snipped fresh dill
½ teaspoon apple cider vinegar

¼ cup soy milk
Olive-oil spray
1 pound flounder fillets

1. Preheat the broiler.

2. Place the garlic in a food processor with the S blade inserted. Mince. Add the tofu, dill, vinegar, and soy milk. Process until smooth.

3. Spray both sides of the flounder fillets with oil. Place the fillets on a broiler pan, glossy side up. Broil for about 3 minutes and turn over. Broil for 3 more minutes.

4. Place the broiled fish on a serving platter and spoon the sauce over the fillets.

PLANT ESTROGEN ESTIMATE: ½ PORTION PER SERVING

BROILED SALMON WITH DIJON SAUCE

Work and Cooking Time: *under 15 minutes*
Equipment: *electric food processor*
Yield: *Makes 4 servings*

Adding this Dijon mustard sauce to salmon makes a doubly healthy high-protein dish.

2 garlic cloves, quartered

2 tablespoons Dijon mustard

2 teaspoons tamari

1 tablespoon lemon juice

½ cake (9½ ounces) silken tofu

½ cup soy milk

Olive-oil spray

4 8-ounce salmon fillets

1. Preheat the broiler.

2. Place the garlic in a food processor with the S blade inserted. Mince. Add the mustard, tamari, lemon juice, tofu, and soy milk. Process until smooth.

3. Spray both sides of the salmon fillets with oil. Place the fillets on a broiler pan, skin side up. Broil for about 3 minutes, until the skin is browned. Turn over and broil for another 3 to 5 minutes, until the fish turns pink all the way through.

4. Place the broiled fish on a serving platter and spoon the sauce over the fillets.

PLANT ESTROGEN ESTIMATE: ¾ PORTION PER SERVING

POACHED COD IN BASIL SAUCE

Work and Cooking Time: *under 15 minutes*
Baking Time: *10 minutes*
Equipment: *electric food processor*
Yield: *Makes 4 servings*

Poached cod smothered in creamy basil sauce makes perfect food for menopause. Cod is a super source of calcium, and the sauce is rich in natural estrogens.

Fish

1 pound cod fillets
3 garlic cloves, quartered
1 bay leaf
Pinch salt and pepper

Sauce

2 garlic cloves, quartered
1 cup fresh basil leaves

½ cake (9½ ounces) silken tofu
½ cup soy milk
1 teaspoon Dijon mustard
1 tablespoon lemon juice
Salt

4 lemon slices

1. Preheat the oven to 400°F.

2. Place the fish in a shallow casserole dish. In a small bowl, combine the garlic, bay leaf, 2 cups of water, salt, and pepper. Pour over the fish. Cover with foil. Place in the oven for 10 minutes, or until cooked through.

3. While the fish poaches, prepare the sauce: Place the garlic in a food processor with the S blade inserted. Mince. Add the basil. Process until well chopped. Add the tofu and soy milk. Process until smooth.

4. Pour into a saucepan; heat over medium heat.

5. When the fish is fully cooked, remove it from the oven. Place the poached fish on a shallow serving dish.

6. Remove the sauce from the burner. Whisk in the mustard and lemon juice. Salt to taste. Taste again. If needed, add more lemon juice and mustard. Spoon over the fish. Garnish with slices of lemon.

PLANT ESTROGEN ESTIMATE: ¾ PORTION PER SERVING

FLOUNDER ON A BED OF CREAMY
CURRIED WATERCRESS

Work and Cooking Time: *under 20 minutes*
Equipment: *electric food processor*
Yield: *Makes 4 servings*

Delicate white fish sprinkled with turmeric on a bed of yellow and green makes a pretty main course. Easy to make and fun to serve, this dish surprises you by its subtle sweet taste.

Any delicate white fish—sole, tilapia, bass, even cod—can be substituted for flounder. Choose young watercress. If the sprigs are tender and less than 4 inches long, you can use stems and all.

1 garlic clove, quartered	1 teaspoon honey
¼ cake (4 ounces) soft tofu	3 cups (4 ounces) young watercress, washed
1½ teaspoons lemon juice	Olive-oil spray
½ teaspoon curry powder	4 4-ounce flounder fillets
¼ teaspoon ground cinnamon	Turmeric
1 tablespoon yellow miso	

1. Preheat the broiler.

2. Place the garlic in a food processor with the S blade inserted. Mince. Add the tofu, lemon juice, curry powder, cinnamon, miso, and honey. Process until smooth and silky. (All graininess should disappear.) Taste. If needed, add more miso. Set aside.

3. Steam the watercress in a steamer over 2 cups of water for 5 minutes or until tender.

4. While the watercress steams, prepare the fish: Spray both sides of the fillets with olive oil. Place the fillets on a broiler pan, shiny side up. Broil for 2 minutes, until white and opaque. Turn the fillets over. Broil for 2 to 3 minutes, until the flesh is white through to the middle. Remove from the oven.

5. Place the steamed watercress in a mixing bowl. Stir in the curried sauce. Place on a serving dish. Lay the fish fillets on top of the watercress curry. Sprinkle with turmeric. Serve.

PLANT ESTROGEN ESTIMATE: ¼ PORTION PER SERVING

COD IN ORANGE-GINGER SAUCE

Work and Cooking Time: *under 10 minutes*
Baking Time: *20 minutes*
Equipment: *electric food processor*
Yield: *Makes 4 servings*

16 ounces cod fillets
2 garlic cloves, quartered
7 ⅛×1-inch slices fresh ginger
3 tablespoons frozen orange juice concentrate

½ teaspoon grated orange rind
1 tablespoon yellow miso
1 cake (19 ounces) silken tofu

1. Preheat the oven to 400°F.

2. Arrange the cod fillets in a baking dish. Pour ½ cup of water over the fish. Cover with foil. Bake for 20 minutes, until a fork easily pierces the fish.

3. While the fish bakes, prepare the sauce: Place the garlic in a food processor with the S blade inserted. Mince. Add the ginger. Mince. Add the orange juice concentrate, orange rind, miso, and tofu. Process until smooth. Pour into a pot; heat without boiling.

4. Remove the cod from the oven. Arrange it on a serving dish. Pour warm sauce over the fillets before serving.

PLANT ESTROGEN ESTIMATE: 1 PORTION PER SERVING

SALMON LOAF WITH WHITE SAUCE

Work Time: *under 10 minutes*
Baking Time: *1 hour*
Equipment: *electric food processor*
Yield: *Makes 6 servings*

An estrogenic rendition of a family favorite. I loved my mother's salmon loaf with white sauce best of all. The bones in canned salmon make it an excellent calcium source.

Loaf

5 garlic cloves, quartered

1 cake (16 ounces) extra-firm tofu

15-ounce can salmon, drained

¼ cup fresh dill

1 tablespoon dill seeds

½ cup chopped scallion

¼ cup flaxseed

¼ cup soy milk

¼ cup bacin bits

White Sauce

3 garlic cloves, quartered

½ cake (9½ ounces) silken tofu

2 tablespoons lemon juice

¼ cup fresh dill

Salt and pepper

1. Preheat the oven to 400°F.

2. Place the garlic in a food processor with the S blade inserted. Mince. Break the tofu into several pieces and place in the food processor. Add the drained salmon, fresh dill, dill seeds, scallion, flaxseed, soy milk, and bacin bits. Process until puréed.

3. Turn into a 9×5-inch nonstick or oiled loaf pan. Bake for 1 hour, until the center is firm and the edges are browned.

4. While the loaf bakes, prepare the sauce: Place the garlic in a food processor with the S blade inserted. Mince. Add the tofu, lemon juice, and dill. Process until smooth. Add salt and pepper to taste.

4. Turn the loaf onto a serving platter. Slice and serve with sauce.

PLANT ESTROGEN ESTIMATE: 1½ PORTIONS PER SERVING

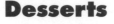

Eleven

Desserts

Finally! Every word, every recipe in this book has been a prelude. Now you get to the substance—*desserts!*

You think I'm joking? I'm not. Desserts are my inspiration and motivation. Ever since I made my first chocolate pudding, I've lain awake at night fantasizing about new sweet treats—mousses, cheesecakes, cookies, pies, ice creams, and more puddings. My menopausal motto is, "A slice of mousse cake a day keeps the hot flashes away."

Let's take a look at these desserts. All the soy desserts—puddings, mousses, cheesecakes, custards, and sauces—are protein-packed, vitamin-rich, calcium-loaded, and estrogen-filled. Most go heavy on fruit and light on sugar. Frozen juice concentrates, all-fruit jams, and dried fruits provide a large portion of the sweetness and flavor. Since minerals are preserved when fruit is condensed into juice concentrates, jams, and dried fruits, these desserts also boost your boron.

All the flaxseed desserts—pie crusts, fruit crisps, cookies, and squares—are made without eggs or oil. Not only are they fabulous sources of plant estrogens, they're excellent sources of omega-3 essential fatty acids. You may do your heart good with these potentially cholesterol-lowering goodies. All in all, these desserts are real food.

So munch away and save room for dessert.

≋ SAUCES

Use these sauces often and everywhere—over pies and crumbles, cakes and custards.

CINNAMON-SESAME SAUCE

≋

Work Time: *under 5 minutes*
Equipment: *electric food processor*
Yield: *Makes about 1 cup*

As quick a dessert sauce as you'll ever make. Whip it up in minutes. Spoon it over fresh berries, fruit pies, baked apples, or cakes. Instantly, any dessert is fancier.

½ cake (9½ ounces) silken tofu

¼ cup soy milk

2 teaspoons tahini

2 tablespoons honey

1 teaspoon lemon extract

1 tablespoon ground cinnamon

Place all of the ingredients in a food processor with the S blade inserted. Process until smooth. Taste. If needed, add more lemon extract or cinnamon. Serve.

PLANT ESTROGEN ESTIMATE: **2¼** PORTIONS PER RECIPE

APPLE-CINNAMON SAUCE

Work Time: *under 5 minutes*
Equipment: *electric food processor*
Yield: *Makes 1 cup*

Another simple sauce to pour over pies and crumbles.

½ cake (9½ ounces) silken tofu
1 teaspoon orange extract
1 teaspoon vanilla extract

1 tablespoon ground cinnamon
2 tablespoons apple butter
¼ cup frozen apple juice concentrate

Place all of the ingredients in a food processor with the S blade inserted. Process until smooth. Taste. If needed, add more orange extract, vanilla, or cinnamon.

PLANT ESTROGEN ESTIMATE: **2** PORTIONS PER RECIPE

CREAMY VANILLA SAUCE

Work Time: *under 5 minutes*
Equipment: *electric food processor*
Yield: *Makes 1 cup*

Use this all-purpose topping on any dessert that screams out for a dab of some sweet, white, creamy stuff—pumpkin pie, walnut pie, or pudding.

½ cake (9½ ounces) silken tofu
¼ cup soy milk
1 tablespoon vanilla extract

3 tablespoons maple syrup
1 teaspoon ground cardamom
1 tablespoon cashew butter

Place all of the ingredients in a food processor with the S blade inserted. Process until smooth and creamy. Taste. If needed, add more vanilla.

PLANT ESTROGEN ESTIMATE: 2¼ PORTIONS PER RECIPE

CREAMY ORANGE SAUCE

Work Time: *under 5 minutes*
Equipment: *electric blender*
Yield: *Makes 1¼ cups*

A vitamin C booster! This sauce gives fruit pies and crisps an orange twist.

½ cake (9½ ounces) silken tofu
⅓ cup frozen orange juice concentrate
¼ cup frozen apple juice concentrate

½ teaspoon orange extract
1 teaspoon vanilla extract
1 tablespoon all-fruit orange marmalade

Place all of the ingredients in an electric blender. Blend until smooth. Taste. If needed, add more orange extract or vanilla.

PLANT ESTROGEN ESTIMATE: 2 PORTIONS PER RECIPE

PEACH SAUCE

Work Time: *under 5 minutes*
Equipment: *electric food processor*
Yield: *Makes ¾ cup*

Pour this sauce over a bowl full of fresh fruit. Violà! Estrogenic fruit salad.

½ cake (9½ ounces) silken tofu
¼ cup all-fruit peach jam
½ cup soy milk

½ teaspoon orange extract
1 tablespoon vanilla extract
½ teaspoon ground cardamom

Place all of the ingredients in a food processor with the S blade inserted. Process until smooth and creamy. Taste. If needed, add more orange extract, vanilla, or cardamom.

PLANT ESTROGEN ESTIMATE: **2½** PORTIONS PER RECIPE

BANANA-STRAWBERRY SAUCE

Work Time: *under 5 minutes*
Equipment: *electric blender*
Yield: *Makes 3½ cups*

Pour on this creamy pink sauce and transform cold cereal into a morning dessert, or fruit salad into a protein-rich meal.

1 cake (19 ounces) silken tofu
1 cup strawberries, fresh or frozen
1 banana, sliced
½ cup soy milk

½ cup frozen white grape juice concentrate
½ teaspoon banana extract
1 teaspoon vanilla extract

Place all of the ingredients in an electric blender. Blend until smooth and creamy. Taste. If needed, add more banana extract or vanilla.

PLANT ESTROGEN ESTIMATE: **4½ PORTIONS PER RECIPE**

≋ PUDDINGS AND CUSTARDS

Creamy desserts without cream! Cut calories. Increase protein. Lower cholesterol. Get plant estrogens. Eat pudding, custard, and mousse for breakfast, lunch, or dinner!

CHOCOLATE VELVET PUDDING

≋

Work Time: *under 5 minutes*
Equipment: *electric food processor*
Yield: *Makes 4 servings*

Chocolate is not a health food, but it is irresistible. So, since most of us are going to eat it anyway, we might as well make it estrogenically rich! This chocolate pudding is not only the easiest pudding you'll ever make, it's also the healthiest form of chocolate you'll ever eat. It's packed with protein, bursting with calcium, and overflowing with plant estrogens.

1 cake (19 ounces) silken tofu
½ cup unsweetened cocoa powder
¼ cup maple syrup

1 tablespoon blackstrap molasses
1 tablespoon vanilla extract

Place all of the ingredients in a food processor with the S blade inserted. Process until smooth and creamy. Taste. If needed, add more vanilla. Spoon into dessert dishes. Serve or refrigerate.

PLANT ESTROGEN ESTIMATE: **1 PORTION PER SERVING**

PEPPERMINT-CHOCOLATE CHIP PUDDING

Work Time: *under 5 minutes*
Equipment: *electric food processor*
Yield: *Makes 4 servings*

Definitely not a health food! Still, if you're going to indulge in chocolate and chocolate chips, at least you'll be adding health-giving soy to your pleasure.

1 cake (19 ounces) silken tofu
⅓ cup unsweetened cocoa powder
¼ cup maple syrup
1 tablespoon blackstrap molasses

1 teaspoon vanilla extract
¼ teaspoon peppermint extract
¼ cup mini chocolate chips

Place the tofu, cocoa powder, maple syrup, molasses, and vanilla and peppermint extracts in a food processor with the S blade inserted. Process until smooth and creamy. Taste. If needed, add more vanilla. Pour into a bowl. Stir in the chocolate chips. Spoon into dessert dishes. Serve or refrigerate.

PLANT ESTROGEN ESTIMATE: **1** PORTION PER SERVING

MAPLE-WALNUT PUDDING

Work Time: *under 5 minutes*
Equipment: *electric food processor*
Yield: *Makes 4 servings*

Another wonderful no-cook pudding packed with healthy natural estrogens!

1 cake (19 ounces) silken tofu
¼ cup maple syrup
¼ cup cashew or almond butter

1 teaspoon maple extract
1 tablespoon vanilla extract
⅓ cup chopped walnuts

Place the tofu, maple syrup, nut butter, maple extract, and vanilla in a food processor with the S blade inserted. Process until smooth and creamy. Taste. If needed, add more vanilla. Pour into a bowl. Stir in the walnuts. Spoon into dessert dishes. Serve or refrigerate.

PLANT ESTROGEN ESTIMATE: 1 PORTION PER SERVING

PUMPKIN CUSTARD

Work Time: *under 10 minutes*
Equipment: *electric food processor*
Yield: *Makes 6 servings*

For a super-quick classic winter dessert, this can't be beat. For extra holiday flair, you can top it with a dab of Cinnamon-Sesame Sauce (page 231).

16-ounce can solid-pack pumpkin pie filling
1 cake (about 19 ounces) silken tofu
⅓ cup maple syrup or brown sugar

2 tablespoons pumpkin pie spice
1 tablespoon vanilla extract
1 tablespoon blackstrap molasses

Place all of the ingredients in a food processor with the S blade inserted. Process until smooth and creamy. Taste. If needed, add more pumpkin pie spice. Spoon into dessert dishes. Serve or refrigerate.

PLANT ESTROGEN ESTIMATE: ¾ PORTION PER SERVING

GAVIN'S TAPIOCA PUDDING

※

Work and Cooking Time: *under 15 minutes*
Yield: *Makes 4 servings*

When my friend Gavin was sick, his temperature spiked to 104°F and he craved only one food—tapioca pudding. But he had a problem: He couldn't digest milk. He asked, "Could you try to make me some tapioca pudding somehow?" I concocted this soy milk–based version. He ate it, literally, by the quart. For a while it was the only food he could digest.

Quick-cooking tapioca ensures you can make this recipe quickly. A good old-fashioned British-style custard powder ensures it will taste great. I use Bird's Custard. You can pick it up right alongside the packaged puddings in most supermarkets.

4 cups soy milk

2 tablespoons quick-cooking tapioca

3 tablespoons maple syrup

1 teaspoon ground cardamom

1 envelope custard powder

1. Pour 3¾ cups of soy milk into a heavy-bottomed saucepan. Sprinkle in the tapioca and wait for 3 minutes. Stir in the maple syrup and cardamom. Heat over medium-high heat, stirring occasionally.

2. In a small bowl, dissolve the custard powder in ¼ cup of soy milk.

3. When the tapioca begins to boil lightly, stir in the dissolved custard. Stir continuously until the mixture has thickened. Remove from the heat. Cool before serving.

PLANT ESTROGEN ESTIMATE: 1 PORTION PER SERVING

INDIAN PUDDING

Work Time: *5 minutes*
Baking Time: *10 minutes*
Equipment: *electric food processor*
Yield: *Makes 4 servings*

Another ever-so-simple, quick version of a classic! The blackstrap molasses and cinnamon make this naturally estrogenic dessert high in calcium.

1 cake (16 ounces) soft tofu
1 tablespoon blackstrap molasses
1 tablespoon ground cinnamon
½ teaspoon ground ginger

½ teaspoon ground nutmeg
1 tablespoon vanilla extract
2 tablespoons frozen apple juice concentrate
2 tablespoons maple syrup

1. Preheat the oven to 400°F.
2. Place all of the ingredients in a food processor with the S blade inserted. Process until smooth and creamy. Taste. If needed, add more cinnamon. Place in a casserole dish and cover. Bake for 10 minutes, until hot.

PLANT ESTROGEN ESTIMATE: 1 PORTION PER SERVING

CARDAMOM CUSTARD WITH MAPLE-NUT SAUCE

Work and Cooking Time: *under 15 minutes*
Chilling Time: *1½ hours*
Equipment: *electric food processor*
Yield: *Makes 4 servings*

I tried to make flan in the refrigerator. I didn't get flan, but I did get a wonderfully rich-feeling, melt-in-your-mouth cardamom custard.

Custard

½ cup soy milk

1 teaspoon ground cardamom

1 envelope (1 tablespoon) unflavored gelatin

2 tablespoons vanilla extract

1 cake (19 ounces) silken tofu

Sauce

3 tablespoons maple syrup

¼ cake (4¾ ounces) silken tofu

1 teaspoon vanilla extract

2 tablespoons chopped walnuts

1. Place the soy milk in a saucepan. Add the cardamom. Sprinkle the gelatin over the soy milk. Place over low heat to dissolve.

2. Place the vanilla and tofu in a food processor with the S blade inserted. Add the dissolved gelatin mixture. Process until smooth and creamy. Taste. If needed, add more cardamom. Pour into four 1-cup gelatin molds. Refrigerate for 1½ hours, until firm. Remove from the molds and place on dessert plates.

3. Prepare the sauce: Place the maple syrup, tofu, and vanilla in a food processor with the S blade inserted. Process until smooth. Taste. If needed, add more vanilla. Stir in the walnuts. Spoon the sauce over the unmolded custards.

PLANT ESTROGEN ESTIMATE: 1¼ PORTIONS PER SERVING

ALMOND-COFFEE CUSTARD

Work Time: *under 5 minutes*
Baking Time: *1 hour*
Equipment: *electric food processor*
Yield: *Makes 3 servings*

Amazing! Baked custard without eggs!

1 cake (19 ounces) silken tofu

¼ cup grain coffee

⅓ cup maple syrup

1 teaspoon almond extract

1. Preheat the oven to 225°F.

2. Place all of the ingredients in a food processor with the S blade inserted. Process until smooth and creamy. Taste. If needed, add more almond extract. Pour into three 8-ounce custard cups.

3. Place the custard cups in a baking dish with ½ inch of water. Bake for 1 hour, until set. Cool before serving.

PLANT ESTROGEN ESTIMATE: 1⅓ PORTIONS PER SERVING

LEMON CUSTARD

Work Time: *under 5 minutes*
Baking Time: *1 hour*
Equipment: *electric food processor*
Yield: *Makes 3 servings*

Be certain to bake this one on low heat. It curdles easily.

1 cake (19 ounces) silken tofu
¼ cup lemon juice
⅓ cup raw sugar

1 teaspoon lemon extract
1 tablespoon vanilla extract

1. Preheat the oven to 225°F.

2. Place all of the ingredients in a food processor with the S blade inserted. Process until smooth and creamy. Taste. If needed, add more lemon extract or vanilla. Pour into three 8-ounce custard cups.

3. Place the custard cups in a baking dish with ½ inch of water. Bake for 1 hour, until set. Cool before serving.

PLANT ESTROGEN ESTIMATE: 1⅓ PORTIONS PER SERVING

NOODLE KUGEL

Work and Cooking Time: *under 15 minutes*
Baking Time: *1½ hours*
Equipment: *electric food processor*
Yield: *Makes 9 servings*

A low-fat, high-protein, no-cholesterol version of a traditional heart-stopper.

6 ounces medium egg noodles

1 cup raisins

2 tablespoons ground cinnamon

1½ teaspoons ground nutmeg

2 tablespoons vanilla extract

⅓ cup maple syrup

1½ cakes (28½ ounces) silken tofu

1. Preheat the oven to 250°F.

2. Bring 6 cups of water to a boil. Place the noodles in the boiling water. Cook for 5 minutes. Drain. Rinse with cool water. Place in a medium-size mixing bowl. Stir in the raisins.

3. Place the remaining ingredients in a food processor with the S blade inserted. Process until smooth and creamy. Pour into the bowl with the noodles and raisins. Stir until combined.

4. Turn into a 9×9-inch nonstick or oiled baking pan. Place this pan in another, larger baking pan. Pour ½ inch of water into the outer pan. Bake for 1½ hours, until the custard sets. Cool. Cut into nine 3-inch squares.

PLANT ESTROGEN ESTIMATE: ⅔ PORTION PER SERVING

TORTES AND CRUMBLES

There's no added fat here. All of these use all-fruit preserves to form a dough—never so much as a pat of butter—and all of these crumbles use malt or syrup to create crunch—never so much as a drop of oil.

QUICK CHERRY CRUMBLE

Work and Cooking Time: *under 20 minutes*
Baking Time: *10 minutes*
Equipment: *electric coffee grinder*
Yield: *Makes 8 servings*

You won't believe this is a quick dessert. The first time you make it, it may take a few extra minutes to follow the directions. By the second time, you'll find this the easiest pie you'll ever make! It's great with Creamy Vanilla Sauce (page 232).

Crumble Topping
¾ cup flaxseed
3 tablespoons chopped walnuts
1 teaspoon ground cardamom
¼ cup maple syrup

Filling
2 16-ounce packages frozen pitted cherries
¾ cup frozen apple juice or white grape juice concentrate
3 tablespoons cornstarch
¼ cup frozen apple juice concentrate, thawed

1. Preheat the oven to 300°F.
2. To prepare the topping, grind the flaxseed in an electric coffee grinder in two batches. Place in a mixing bowl. Add the nuts, cardamom, and maple syrup. Mix thoroughly. Spread on a cookie sheet. Bake for 5 minutes. Remove from the oven and stir with a spatula. Bake for 5 more minutes, until toasted.
3. While the crumble topping bakes, prepare the filling: Place the frozen cherries and frozen juice concentrate in a pot. Cover and cook over medium-high heat. Dissolve the cornstarch in the ¼ cup of thawed juice concentrate. Stir it into the cooking fruit. Continue stirring until the mixture thickens and becomes translucent. Remove from the heat. Pour into a 9-inch pie plate.
4. Spoon the crumble over the fruit. Serve warm or cold.

PLANT ESTROGEN ESTIMATE: 1½ PORTIONS PER SERVING

QUICK RHUBARB CRUMBLE

≋

Work and Cooking Time: *under 20 minutes*
Baking Time: *10 minutes*
Equipment: *electric coffee grinder*
Yield: *Makes 6 servings*

This simple crumble provides a way to appreciate rhubarb when it's in season *and* get your estrogen. Try it with Creamy Vanilla Sauce (page 232).

Crumble Topping
¾ cup flaxseed
¼ cup chopped walnuts
¼ cup maple syrup
1 tablespoon vanilla extract

Filling
1 cup frozen apple juice concentrate
6 cups sliced rhubarb
¼ cup cornstarch
¼ cup maple syrup

1. Preheat the oven to 300°F.

2. To prepare the topping, grind the flaxseed in an electric coffee grinder in two batches. Place in a mixing bowl. Add the nuts, maple syrup, and vanilla. Mix thoroughly. Spread on a cookie sheet. Bake for 5 minutes. Remove from the oven and stir with a spatula. Bake for 5 more minutes, until toasted.

3. While the crumble topping bakes, prepare the filling: Place the apple juice concentrate in a heavy-bottomed 2-quart saucepan. Add the rhubarb. Cook over medium-high heat for 10 to 15 minutes, until the rhubarb is soft. Dissolve the cornstarch in the maple syrup. Stir the dissolved cornstarch into the cooked rhubarb. Stir continuously until the filling thickens. Remove from the heat. Pour into a 9-inch pie plate.

4. Spoon the crumble over the fruit. Serve warm or cold.

PLANT ESTROGEN ESTIMATE: **2** PORTIONS PER SERVING

QUICK APPLE CRUMBLE

Work and Cooking Time: *under 20 minutes*
Baking Time: *10 minutes*
Equipment: *electric coffee grinder*
Yield: *Makes 6 servings*

Apple crumble in minutes! This nontraditional wonder is great with a slice of cheddar or Creamy Orange Sauce (see page 233).

Crumble Topping
¾ cup flaxseed
¼ cup chopped walnuts or almonds
¼ cup maple syrup
2 teaspoons ground cinnamon
1 teaspoon grated orange rind

Filling
5 apples, grated (don't peel)
1 tablespoon frozen apple juice concentrate
1 tablespoon frozen orange juice concentrate
2 teaspoons grated orange peel
2 teaspoons ground cinnamon
1 tablespoon cornstarch
¼ cup raisins

1. Preheat the oven to 300°F.

2. To prepare the topping, grind the flaxseed in an electric coffee grinder in two batches. Place in a mixing bowl. Add the nuts, maple syrup, cinnamon, and orange rind. Mix thoroughly. Spread on a cookie sheet. Bake for 5 minutes. Remove from the oven and stir with a spatula. Bake for 5 more minutes, until toasted.

3. While the crumble topping bakes, prepare the filling: Place all of the filling ingredients in a heavy-bottomed pot. Mix until the apple is thoroughly combined with the flavorings and cornstarch. Cook over medium-high heat, stirring occasionally, until the apple is heated and a sauce has formed. Remove from the heat. Pour into a 9-inch pie plate.

4. Spoon the crumble over the fruit. Serve warm or cold.

PLANT ESTROGEN ESTIMATE: **2** PORTIONS PER SERVING

STRAWBERRY-RHUBARB CRUMBLE

Work Time: *under 15 minutes*
Baking Time: *30 minutes*
Equipment: *electric coffee grinder*
Yield: *Makes 8 servings*

I made this one for my fiftieth birthday. It was a hit.

Filling
1 quart fresh strawberries, sliced
3 cups sliced rhubarb
½ cup maple syrup
¼ cup all-fruit strawberry jam
¼ cup flaxseed

Crumble Topping
⅔ cup flaxseed
⅓ cup chopped walnuts
⅓ cup soy flour
2 tablespoons maple syrup
3 tablespoons all-fruit strawberry jam

1. Preheat the oven to 325°F.

2. To prepare the filling, place the strawberries and rhubarb in a large mixing bowl. Stir in the maple syrup and jam, coating the fruit. Grind the flaxseed in an electric coffee grinder. Stir into the fruit mixture, distributing the ground seeds throughout. Pour into an 11-inch pie plate.

3. To prepare the topping, grind the flaxseed in an electric coffee grinder ⅓ cup at a time. Pour into a medium-size mixing bowl. Stir in the nuts and soy flour. Add the maple syrup and jam. Mix thoroughly. Spoon the crumble over the filling.

4. Bake for 30 minutes, until the rhubarb is soft and the crumble is lightly browned..

PLANT ESTROGEN ESTIMATE: **2** PORTIONS PER SERVING

RHUBARB CUSTARD CRUMBLE

Work and Cooking Time: *under 25 minutes*
Baking Time: *2 hours*
Equipment: *electric food processor and electric coffee grinder*
Yield: *Makes 8 servings*

Another invention for my fiftieth birthday.

Custard
3 cups sliced rhubarb
¼ cup unbleached white flour
½ cup maple syrup
1 cake (19 ounces) silken tofu
½ cup all-fruit strawberry jam
1 tablespoon vanilla extract

Crumble Topping
⅔ cup flaxseed
¼ cup chopped walnuts
⅓ cup soy flour
½ cup brown rice syrup
3 tablespoons all-fruit strawberry jam

1. Preheat the oven to 225°F.

2. Place the rhubarb in a medium-size mixing bowl. Add the flour and maple syrup. Stir, coating the rhubarb with flour and syrup. Pour into a 12-inch pie plate.

3. Place the tofu, jam, and vanilla in a food processor with the S blade inserted. Process until smooth and creamy. Pour over the rhubarb. Spread evenly.

4. To prepare the topping, grind the flaxseed in an electric coffee grinder ⅓ cup at a time. Pour into a medium-size mixing bowl. Stir in the nuts and soy flour. Pour the rice syrup into a small pan. Boil for 1 minute. Add to the flaxseed mixture, along with the jam. Mix thoroughly. Spoon the crumble over the custard layer.

5. Bake for 2 hours, until the rhubarb is soft and the crumble is lightly browned.

PLANT ESTROGEN ESTIMATE: 2⅓ PORTIONS PER SERVING

STRAWBERRY-KIWI TORTE

Work and Cooking Time: *under 20 minutes*
Baking Time: *10 minutes*
Equipment: *electric coffee grinder and electric food processor*
Yield: *Makes 6 servings*

Looks and tastes like summertime. Feel free to substitute any brightly colored summer fruit or berries.

Glaze

⅓ cup all-fruit apricot jam
3 tablespoons frozen apple juice concentrate, thawed
½ teaspoon unflavored gelatin

Crust

⅔ cup flaxseed
⅔ cup soy flour
½ cup chopped walnuts
⅓ cup all-fruit apricot jam

Topping

½ cake (8 ounces) soft tofu
3 tablespoons all-fruit apricot jam
1 tablespoon vanilla extract
½ teaspoon lemon extract
½ teaspoon almond extract
1 pint fresh strawberries, hulled and halved
1 kiwi, peeled and sliced

1. Preheat the oven to 350°F.

2. To prepare the glaze, whisk the apricot jam and apple juice concentrate together. Sprinkle the gelatin over the mixture. While the gelatin is absorbed, prepare the crust and filling.

3. To prepare the crust, grind the flaxseed in an electric coffee grinder ⅓ cup at a time. Pour the ground seeds into a small mixing bowl. Add the soy flour and nuts. Stir until well combined. Mix in the jam to form a dough. Turn into a 10-inch nonstick or oiled torte pan. Press evenly over the bottom and up the sides. Bake for 10 minutes, until lightly browned. Remove from the oven to cool.

4. While the crust cools, prepare the topping: Place the tofu, jam, vanilla, lemon extract, and almond extract in a food processor with the S blade inserted. Process until smooth. Taste. If needed, add more lemon or almond extract. Spread in a thin, even layer

over the baked crust. Arrange the halved strawberries and sliced kiwi in concentric circles on top of the creamy filling.

5. Heat the glaze until it is warm and the gelatin has dissolved. Spoon a light layer evenly over the fruit. Refrigerate until the glaze sets. Serve.

PLANT ESTROGEN ESTIMATE: 2½ PORTIONS PER SERVING

APPLE TORTE

Work Time: *under 15 minutes*
Baking Time: *30 minutes*
Equipment: *electric coffee grinder*
Yield: *Makes 6 servings*

A crusty, nutty fruit dessert. Wonderful topped with Cinnamon Sesame Sauce (page 231).

Crust
⅔ cup flaxseed
⅔ cup soy flour
⅓ cup chopped almonds
½ cup all-fruit orange marmalade

Glaze
¼ cup all-fruit orange marmalade
1 tablespoon frozen apple juice concentrate

Topping
2 apples, halved, cored, and sliced thin
1 teaspoon ground cinnamon
1 tablespoon frozen apple juice concentrate

1. Preheat the oven to 350°F.

2. To prepare the crust, grind the flaxseed in an electric coffee grinder ⅓ cup at a time. Pour the ground seeds into a small mixing bowl. Add the soy flour and nuts. Stir until well combined. Mix in the marmalade to form a dough. Turn into a 9-inch nonstick or oiled torte pan. Press evenly over the bottom and up the sides.

3. To prepare the topping, place the sliced apples, cinnamon, and apple juice concentrate in a mixing bowl. Toss to coat the apples. Arrange the apple slices in concentric circles, covering the crust. Bake for 30 minutes, until the crust is light brown and the apples are soft.

4. To prepare the glaze, whisk the marmalade and apple juice concentrate together. Spoon a light layer of glaze evenly over the fruit. Serve.

PLANT ESTROGEN ESTIMATE: 1⅚ PORTIONS PER SERVING

PECAN TORTE

Work and Cooking Time: *under 15 minutes*
Baking Time: *40 minutes*
Equipment: *electric coffee grinder*
Yield: *Makes 6 servings*

A pecan pie without oil or sugar! It's great with Creamy Vanilla Sauce (page 232).

Crust
½ cup flaxseed
½ cup soy flour
⅓ cup all-fruit strawberry jam

Topping
¾ cup frozen white grape juice concentrate
⅓ cup flaxseed
3 tablespoons vanilla extract
¼ cup all-fruit peach jam
1½ cups shelled pecan halves

1. Preheat the oven to 300°F.
2. To prepare the crust, grind the flaxseed in an electric coffee grinder. Pour the ground seeds into a small mixing bowl. Add the soy flour. Stir until well combined. Mix in the jam to form a dough. Turn into a 9-inch nonstick or oiled torte pan. Press evenly over the bottom and up the sides. Bake for 10 minutes.

3. To prepare the topping, heat the juice concentrate to simmering. Grind the flaxseed to a fine meal in an electric coffee grinder. Remove the juice from the heat. Whisk in the ground flaxseed, vanilla, and jam.

4. Remove the crust from the oven. Distribute the pecans evenly over the crust. Spoon the flaxseed mixture over the pecans. Bake for 30 minutes, until the topping has set. Cool. Serve.

PLANT ESTROGEN ESTIMATE: 2⅓ PORTIONS PER SERVING

≋ CHEESECAKES

Extra-firm tofu makes the best New York–style cheesecakes, but patience is required. You have to purée the tofu in your food processor for a full 5 minutes. The noise of the machine grates on the nerves, so turn it on, leave the room, and come back when the work is done.

ORANGE CHEESECAKE

≋

Work Time: *under 20 minutes*
Baking Time: *35 minutes*
Chilling Time: *30 minutes*
Equipment: *electric coffee grinder and electric food processor*
Yield: *Makes 6 servings*

Somewhere between cake-like and cream-like, this orange cheesecake resembles New York–style cheesecake.

Crust
⅓ cup flaxseed
¼ cup soy flour
¼ cup chopped walnuts or almonds
¼ cup all-fruit orange marmalade

Filling
1 cake (16 ounces) extra-firm tofu
½ cup frozen orange juice concentrate
3 tablespoons maple syrup
1 tablespoon vanilla extract
½ teaspoon orange extract

Glaze

½ cup all-fruit orange marmalade

1. Preheat the oven to 400°F.

2. To make the crust, grind the flaxseed to a fine meal using an electric coffee grinder. Pour the ground seeds into a small mixing bowl. Stir in the soy flour and nuts. Add the marmalade. Blend with a spoon to form a dough. Press the dough into a nonstick or oiled 7-inch springform pan, covering the bottom evenly. Bake for 5 minutes.

3. To prepare the filling, break the tofu into about eight pieces and place them in a food processor with the S blade inserted. Add the orange juice concentrate, maple syrup, vanilla, and orange extract. Process for 5 minutes, until completely smooth. Taste. If needed, add more vanilla or orange extract. Pour the filling into the springform pan. Bake for 30 minutes, or until the middle of the cheesecake has set.

4. To glaze, spoon a thin layer of marmalade over the cheesecake. Chill the cheesecake for 30 minutes. Run a knife around the outer edge of cake. Remove the pan. Serve.

PLANT ESTROGEN ESTIMATE: 1⅔ PORTIONS PER SERVING

LEMON-POPPY SEED CHEESECAKE

Work Time: *under 20 minutes*
Baking Time: *35 minutes*
Chilling Time: *30 minutes*
Equipment: *electric coffee grinder and electric food processor*
Yield: *Makes 6 servings*

Poppy seeds are worth eating. They're higher in calcium than any other food on the nutrition charts. When you eat this estrogen-rich cheesecake, you cash in on a calcium sweepstakes.

Crust

3 tablespoons flaxseed

3 tablespoons soy flour

3 tablespoons poppy seeds

2 tablespoons orange marmalade

1 tablespoon frozen apple juice concentrate

Filling

1 cake (16 ounces) extra-firm tofu

½ cup all-fruit orange marmalade

⅓ cup lemon juice

¼ cup maple syrup

½ cup poppy seeds

1 teaspoon ground cardamom

1 tablespoon lemon extract

1. Preheat the oven to 400°F.

2. To make the crust, grind the flaxseed to a fine meal using an electric coffee grinder. Pour the ground seeds into a small mixing bowl. Stir in the soy flour and poppy seeds. Add the marmalade and apple juice concentrate. Blend with a spoon to form a dough. Press the dough into a nonstick or oiled 7-inch springform pan, covering the bottom evenly. Bake for 5 minutes.

3. To prepare the filling, break the tofu into about eight pieces and place them in a food processor with the S blade inserted. Add the remaining filling ingredients. Process for 5 minutes, until completely smooth. Taste. If needed, add more cardamom. Pour the filling into the springform pan. Bake for 30 minutes, or until the middle of the cheesecake has set.

4. Chill the cheesecake for 30 minutes. Run a knife around the outer edge of the cake. Remove the pan. Serve.

PLANT ESTROGEN ESTIMATE: 1¼ PORTIONS PER SERVING

≋ MOUSSES AND MOUSSE CAKES

Gelatin and silken tofu make cream-free, eggless mousse and mousse cake possible. These cholesterol-cutting estrogenic marvels are my favorite foods.

ORANGE MOUSSE CAKE

Work and Cooking Time: *under 15 minutes*
Baking Time: *10 minutes*
Chilling Time: *2½ hours*
Equipment: *electric coffee grinder and electric food processor*
Yield: *Makes 6 servings*

A very light and creamy way to get your vitamin C, protein, and plant estrogens.

Summer alert! When the weather is hot and humid, this recipe will require an additional ½ teaspoon of gelatin in the filling. Without more gelatin, the cake will not hold its shape.

Crust
¼ cup flaxseed
¼ cup soy flour
¼ cup chopped walnuts
3 tablespoons all-fruit orange marmalade

Filling
½ cup frozen orange juice concentrate, thawed
1 envelope (1 tablespoon) unflavored gelatin

1 cake (19 ounces) silken tofu
3 tablespoons maple syrup
1 tablespoon vanilla extract
1 teaspoon orange extract

Glaze
½ cup all-fruit orange marmalade
2 tablespoons frozen apple juice concentrate, thawed
½ teaspoon unflavored gelatin

1. Preheat the oven to 350°F.

2. To prepare the crust, grind the flaxseed in an electric coffee grinder. Pour the ground seeds into a small bowl. Add the soy flour, nuts, and marmalade. Blend with a spoon to form a dough. Press the dough into a nonstick or oiled 7-inch springform pan, covering the bottom evenly. Bake for 10 minutes.

3. To prepare the filling, pour the orange juice concentrate into a small saucepan. Sprinkle the gelatin over the juice concentrate. Stir over low heat until dissolved.

4. Place the tofu, maple syrup, vanilla, and orange extract in an electric food processor with the S blade inserted. Add the dissolved gelatin. Process until smooth and creamy. Taste. If needed, add more vanilla. Pour the filling over the baked crust. Chill for 2 hours, until firm.

5. While the cake sets, prepare the glaze: Combine the orange marmalade and juice concentrate in a saucepan. Sprinkle with gelatin. When the gelatin is absorbed, stir over low heat until dissolved. Spread the glaze over the gelled mousse cake. Return to the refrigerator for 30 minutes, until the glaze has set. Run a knife around the outer edge of the cake. Remove the pan. Serve.

PLANT ESTROGEN ESTIMATE: 1½ PORTIONS PER SERVING

CHOCOLATE MOUSSE CAKE WITH RASPBERRY SAUCE

Work and Cooking Time: *under 15 minutes*
Baking Time: *10 minutes*
Chilling Time: *2 hours*
Equipment: *electric coffee grinder, electric food processor, and electric blender*
Yield: *Makes 12 servings*

Not for the daily diet; this is a pure indulgence.

Warm-weather warning! When the temperature is hot, this mousse cake requires an additional teaspoon of unflavored gelatin to maintain its form.

Crust
½ cup flaxseed
⅓ cup soy flour
3 tablespoons unsweetened cocoa powder
½ cup chopped walnuts
1 tablespoon vanilla extract
3 tablespoons all-fruit cherry jam

Filling
⅔ cup frozen apple juice concentrate, thawed
2 envelopes (2 tablespoons) unflavored gelatin
2 cakes (38 ounces) silken tofu

½ cup maple syrup
⅔ cup unsweetened cocoa powder
1 tablespoon vanilla extract
2 teaspoons blackstrap molasses

Sauce
1 pint raspberries, fresh or frozen
⅓ cup all-fruit raspberry jam
1 cup frozen apple juice or white grape juice concentrate, thawed

1. Preheat the oven to 350°F.

2. To prepare the crust, grind the flaxseed in an electric coffee grinder. Pour the ground seeds into a small bowl. Add the soy flour, cocoa powder, nuts, vanilla, and jam. Blend with a spoon to form a dough. Press the dough into a nonstick or oiled 10-inch springform pan, covering the bottom evenly. Bake for 10 minutes.

3. To prepare the filling, pour the apple juice concentrate into a small saucepan. Sprinkle the gelatin over the juice concentrate. Stir over low heat until dissolved.

4. Place the tofu, maple syrup, cocoa powder, vanilla, and molasses in a food processor with the S blade inserted. Add the dissolved gelatin. Process until smooth. Taste. If needed, add more cocoa powder and maple syrup. Pour the filling over the baked crust. Chill for 2 hours, until firm. Run a knife around the outer edge of the cake. Remove the pan.

5. To prepare the raspberry sauce, put all of the sauce ingredients in an electric blender. Blend until smooth. Spoon over individual slices of mousse cake.

PLANT ESTROGEN ESTIMATE: 1½ PORTIONS PER SERVING

CHERRY MOUSSE CAKE

Work and Cooking Time: *under 20 minutes*
Baking Time: *10 minutes*
Chilling Time: *2½ hours*
Equipment: *electric coffee grinder and electric food processor*
Yield: *Makes 8 servings*

A melt-in-your-mouth creamy cake.

Summertime alert! When the temperature and the humidity peak, the filling will need an additional teaspoon of unflavored gelatin.

Crust

⅓ cup flaxseed

¼ cup soy flour

¼ cup chopped almonds

3 tablespoons all-fruit cherry jam

Glaze

¾ cup all-fruit cherry preserves

3 tablespoons frozen grape juice concentrate, thawed

½ teaspoon unflavored gelatin

Mousse

⅓ cup frozen apple juice concentrate, thawed

2 envelopes (2 tablespoons) unflavored gelatin

1 cake (19 ounces) silken tofu

⅓ cup all-fruit cherry jam

1 teaspoon vanilla extract

1 teaspoon lemon extract

16 ounces frozen pitted cherries, thawed and drained

1. Preheat the oven to 350°F.

2. To prepare the crust, grind the flaxseed in an electric coffee grinder. Pour the ground seeds into a small bowl. Add the soy flour, nuts, and jam. Blend with a spoon to form a dough. Press the dough into a nonstick or oiled 10-inch springform pan, covering the bottom evenly. Bake for 10 minutes.

3. To prepare the filling, pour the apple juice concentrate into a small saucepan. Sprinkle the gelatin over the juice concentrate. Stir over low heat until dissolved.

4. Place the tofu, jam, vanilla, and lemon extract in a food processor with the S blade inserted. Add the dissolved gelatin. Process until smooth. Taste. If needed, add more vanilla or lemon extract. Pour into a bowl. Stir in the cherries. Pour the filling over the baked crust. Chill for 2 hours, until firm.

5. While the cake sets, prepare the glaze: Mix the cherry preserves and grape juice concentrate in a small saucepan. Sprinkle with gelatin. When the gelatin is absorbed, stir over low heat until dissolved. Spread the glaze over the surface of the cake. Return to the refrigerator for 30 minutes, until the glaze has set. Run a knife around the outer edge of the cake. Remove the pan. Serve.

PLANT ESTROGEN ESTIMATE: 1⅓ PORTIONS PER SERVING

CHOCOLATE-ORANGE MOUSSE CAKE

Work and Cooking Time: *under 20 minutes*
Baking Time: *15 minutes*
Chilling Time: *2 hours*
Equipment: *electric coffee grinder and electric food processor*
Yield: *Makes 6 servings*

Try serving this one with Creamy Orange Sauce (page 233).

Hot-weather warning! When the weather heats up, you'll need to add an additional ½ teaspoon of unflavored gelatin to the filling. Without the extra gelatin, the mousse will not hold its form.

Crust
⅓ cup soy flour
⅓ cup chopped walnuts
2 tablespoons unsweetened cocoa powder
½ cup flaxseed
½ cup all-fruit orange marmalade

Filling
½ cup frozen orange juice concentrate,
  thawed
1 envelope (1 tablespoon) unflavored gelatin
1 cake (19 ounces) silken tofu
¼ cup all-fruit orange marmalade
1 teaspoon orange extract
¼ cup unsweetened cocoa powder
2 tablespoons raw sugar

1. Preheat the oven to 325°F.

2. To prepare the crust, combine the soy flour, nuts, and cocoa in a small mixing bowl. Grind the flaxseed in an electric coffee grinder. Stir the ground seeds into the other dry ingredients. Add the marmalade. Blend with a spoon to form a dough. Press the dough into a nonstick or oiled 7-inch springform pan, lining the entire pan, including the sides. Bake for 15 minutes, until firm and lightly browned.

3. To prepare the filling, pour the orange juice concentrate into a small saucepan. Sprinkle the gelatin over the juice concentrate. Stir over low heat until dissolved.

4. Place the tofu, marmalade, orange extract, cocoa, and sugar in a food processor with the S blade inserted. Add the dissolved gelatin. Process until smooth. Pour the filling over the baked crust. Chill for 2 hours, until firm. Run a knife around the outer edge of the cake. Remove the pan. Serve.

PLANT ESTROGEN ESTIMATE: 1½ PORTIONS PER SERVING

PEAR MOUSSE PIE

Work and Cooking Time: *under 20 minutes*
Baking Time: *10 minutes*
Chilling Time: *2 hours*
Equipment: *electric coffee grinder and electric food processor*
Yield: *Makes 8 servings*

In winter, when fresh fruit is hard to find, I'm grateful for canned pears packed in fruit juice.

Crust
⅔ cup flaxseed
⅔ cup soy flour
⅓ cup chopped walnuts
⅓ cup all-fruit peach jam

Filling
29-ounce can sliced pears in juice
1 envelope (1 tablespoon) unflavored gelatin
1 cake (19 ounces) silken tofu
1 teaspoon cashew butter
1 teaspoon almond extract

1. Preheat the oven to 350°F.

2. To prepare the crust, grind the flaxseed in an electric coffee grinder ⅓ cup at a time. Place the ground seeds in a small mixing bowl. Add the soy flour, nuts, and jam. Blend with a spoon to form a dough. Press the dough into an 11-inch nonstick or oiled pie plate. Cover the bottom and sides of the plate. Bake for 10 minutes.

3. To prepare the filling, drain the pears, reserving ½ cup of juice, and place them in a medium-size mixing bowl. Place the reserved juice in a small saucepan. Sprinkle the gelatin over the juice. Stir over low heat until dissolved.

4. Place the tofu, cashew butter, and almond extract in a food processor with the S blade inserted. Add the dissolved gelatin. Process until smooth. Taste. If needed, add more almond extract. Pour the mixture into the bowl with the pears. Combine. Pour into the baked pie shell. Chill for 2 hours, until firm. Serve.

> PLANT ESTROGEN ESTIMATE: 2¼ PORTIONS PER SERVING

RASPBERRY MOUSSE

Work and Cooking Time: *under 15 minutes*
Chilling Time: *1 hour*
Equipment: *electric food processor*
Yield: *Makes 4 servings*

Especially pretty served in wineglasses or parfait glasses, the light-pink mousse contrasts with the bright-pink topping.

Warm-weather suggestion: In summer, add an additional ½ teaspoon of unflavored gelatin to prevent your mousse from becoming too loose.

Mousse
½ cup frozen apple juice concentrate, thawed
1 envelope (1 tablespoon) unflavored gelatin
12 ounces fresh or frozen raspberries, thawed
2 tablespoons all-fruit raspberry jam
1 teaspoon vanilla extract
1 teaspoon lemon extract
1 cake (19 ounces) silken tofu

Topping
¼ cup all-fruit raspberry jam
2 tablespoons frozen apple juice concentrate

1. Pour the apple juice concentrate into a small saucepan. Sprinkle the gelatin over the juice concentrate. Stir over low heat until dissolved.

2. Place the raspberries, jam, vanilla, lemon extract, and tofu in a food processor with the S blade inserted. Add the dissolved gelatin. Process until smooth and creamy. Taste. If needed, add more vanilla or lemon extract. Spoon into four dessert dishes. Chill until set, about 1 hour.

3. To make the topping, place the jam and juice concentrate in a food processor with the S blade inserted. Process. Spoon a thin layer over the mousse. Serve.

> PLANT ESTROGEN ESTIMATE: 1 PORTION PER SERVING

≋ COOKIES AND BROWNIES

How do brownies get that chewy texture? Lots of oil and eggs, that's how. How do cookies get that crunch? Butter, that's how. How can you get chewy brownies without oil or eggs? Flaxseed. How can you get crunchy cookies without butter or oil? Flaxseed. Try these recipes. You'll be astounded.

CHEWY DATE-NUT SQUARES

≋

Work Time: *under 10 minutes*
Baking Time: *25 minutes*
Equipment: *electric blender and electric coffee grinder*
Yield: *Makes 9 servings*

Very moist and chewy.

⅔ cup whole-wheat pastry flour
⅓ cup soy flour
⅓ cup raw sugar
1½ teaspoons baking powder
½ teaspoon ground nutmeg
½ teaspoon grated orange rind

⅓ cup soy milk
⅔ cup barley malt
½ cup flaxseed
½ cup chopped dates
¼ cup chopped walnuts

1. Preheat the oven to 325°F.

2. Place the whole-wheat flour, soy flour, sugar, baking powder, nutmeg, and orange rind in a medium-size mixing bowl. Stir with a wire whisk until thoroughly combined.

3. Place the soy milk and malt in an electric blender. Grind the flaxseed in an electric coffee grinder ¼ cup at a time. Add to the blender. Blend until thoroughly combined.

4. Pour the liquid mixture into the dry ingredients. Add the dates and walnuts. Stir until combined. Pour the batter into a 9×9-inch nonstick or oiled baking pan. Bake for 25 minutes, until lightly browned around the edges. Cool. Cut into nine 3-inch squares to serve.

PLANT ESTROGEN ESTIMATE: 1 PORTION PER SERVING

BROWNIES

Work Time: *under 15 minutes*
Baking Time: *25 minutes*
Equipment: *electric blender and electric coffee grinder*
Yield: *Makes 9 servings*

A chewy version of the classic American brownie.

⅔ cup whole-wheat pastry flour
½ cup soy flour
¾ cup unsweetened cocoa powder
¾ cup sugar
1½ teaspoons baking powder

⅓ cup soy milk
1 cup barley malt
1 tablespoon vanilla extract
⅔ cup flaxseed

1. Preheat the oven to 325°F.

2. Place the whole-wheat flour, soy flour, cocoa powder, sugar, and baking powder in a medium-size mixing bowl. Stir with a wire whisk until thoroughly combined.

3. Place the soy milk, barley malt, and vanilla in an electric blender. Grind the flaxseed in an electric coffee grinder ⅓ cup at a time. Add to the blender. Blend until all of the ingredients are thoroughly combined and the mixture begins to bubble.

4. Pour the liquid mixture into the dry ingredients. Stir until combined. Pour the batter into a 9×9-inch nonstick or oiled baking pan. Bake for 25 minutes, until the edges are browned and the middle springs back to the touch. Cool. Cut into nine 3-inch squares to serve.

PLANT ESTROGEN ESTIMATE: 1½ PORTIONS PER SERVING

GINGERBREAD

Work Time: *under 15 minutes*
Baking Time: *40 minutes*
Equipment: *electric blender and electric coffee grinder*
Yield: *Makes 9 servings*

Very gingery. Perfectly moist.

1 cup whole-wheat flour	½ teaspoon ground nutmeg
½ cup soy flour	1 cup table molasses
2 teaspoons baking powder	2 tablespoons blackstrap molasses
1 tablespoon ground ginger	1 cup soy milk
1 tablespoon ground cinnamon	1 cup flaxseed

1. Preheat the oven to 325°F.

2. Place the whole-wheat flour, soy flour, baking powder, ginger, cinnamon, and nutmeg in a medium-size mixing bowl. Stir with a wire whisk until thoroughly combined.

3. Place the table molasses, blackstrap molasses, and soy milk in an electric blender. Grind the flaxseed in an electric coffee grinder ⅓ cup at a time. Add to the blender. Blend until all of the ingredients are thoroughly combined and the mixture begins to bubble.

4. Pour the liquid mixture into the dry ingredients. Stir until combined. Pour the batter into a 9×9-inch nonstick or oiled baking pan. Bake for 40 minutes, until the edges are browned. Cool. Cut into nine 3-inch squares to serve.

PLANT ESTROGEN ESTIMATE: **2** PORTIONS PER SERVING

GINGER SNAPS

Work Time: *under 15 minutes*
Baking Time: *1 hour*
Equipment: *electric coffee grinder*
Yield: *Makes 12 cookies*

The longest-baking cookies ever. In the end these come out very crisp—really snappy.

½ cup flaxseed
⅔ cup raw sugar
1 cup unbleached white flour
¼ cup soy flour
1 teaspoon baking powder

1 teaspoon ground cinnamon
2 teaspoons ground ginger
½ cup soy milk
¼ cup table molasses

1. Preheat the oven to 300°F.

2. Grind the flaxseed in an electric coffee grinder ¼ cup at a time. Pour the ground seeds into a medium-size mixing bowl. Add all of the dry ingredients. Stir with a wire whisk until thoroughly combined. Add the soy milk and molasses. Stir with a spoon to make a thick, almost doughlike batter.

3. Spoon heaping tablespoons of cookie dough onto a nonstick or oiled cookie sheet. Using a dampened glass tumbler, flatten each mound. Bake for 1 hour, until lightly browned. Remove from the cookie sheet to cool.

PLANT ESTROGEN ESTIMATE: ¾ PORTION PER COOKIE

LEMON LACE COOKIES

Work Time: *under 15 minutes*
Baking Time: *30 minutes*
Equipment: *electric blender and electric coffee grinder*
Yield: *Makes 24 cookies*

Delicate and crunchy—you won't believe they contain no butter.

⅔ cup unbleached white flour
½ cup soy flour
½ cup raw sugar
1½ tablespoons grated lemon rind
1 teaspoon baking powder
1 teaspoon baking soda

⅔ cup lemon juice
⅔ cup brown rice syrup
1 tablespoon vanilla extract
2 tablespoons lemon extract
⅔ cup flaxseed

1. Preheat the oven to 325°F.

2. Place the unbleached flour, soy flour, sugar, lemon rind, baking powder, and baking soda in a medium-size mixing bowl. Stir with a wire whisk until thoroughly combined.

3. Place the lemon juice, rice syrup, vanilla extract, and lemon extract in an electric blender. Grind the flaxseed in an electric coffee grinder ⅓ cup at a time and pour into the blender. Blend until the mixture bubbles. Pour the liquid mixture into the dry ingredients. Stir until combined.

4. Spoon 2-tablespoon-size mounds of cookie batter onto a well-oiled cookie sheet. Place only eight evenly spaced cookies on a sheet. Bake until the edges of the cookies are lightly browned, about 30 minutes. Remove the cookies from the sheet to cool.

PLANT ESTROGEN ESTIMATE: ½ PORTION PER COOKIE

OATMEAL-RAISIN COOKIES

Work Time: *under 15 minutes*
Baking Time: *30 minutes*
Equipment: *electric blender*
Yield: *Makes 8 cookies*

Huge, moist, old-fashioned cookies.

1 cup rolled oats
¼ cup whole-wheat pastry flour
¼ cup soy flour
½ cup raw sugar
2 teaspoons baking powder
1 teaspoon ground cinnamon
½ teaspoon ground nutmeg

¼ cup table molasses
¾ cup soy milk
½ cup flaxseed
1 tablespoon vanilla extract
½ cup raisins
¼ cup chopped walnuts

1. Preheat the oven to 325°F.

2. Place the rolled oats, whole-wheat pastry flour, soy flour, sugar, baking powder, cinnamon, and nutmeg in a medium-size mixing bowl. Stir with a wire whisk until thoroughly combined.

3. Place the molasses, soy milk, flaxseed, and vanilla in an electric blender. Blend until the seeds disintegrate and the mixture bubbles. Pour the liquid mixture into the dry ingredients. Add the raisins and nuts. Stir to form a cookie batter.

4. Spoon eight mounds of batter onto a nonstick or oiled cookie sheet. Flatten the mounds with a spatula to form large cookies. Bake for 30 minutes, until lightly browned.

SOFT CHOCOLATE COOKIES

Work Time: *under 15 minutes*
Baking Time: *15 minutes*
Equipment: *electric coffee grinder*
Yield: *Makes 16 cookies*

Like a small, round, cakelike brownie.

½ cup flaxseed
⅔ cup whole-wheat pastry flour
¾ cup raw sugar
⅓ cup soy flour
⅓ cup unsweetened cocoa powder

2 teaspoons baking powder
¾ cup soy milk
1 tablespoon blackstrap molasses
1 teaspoon vanilla extract

1. Preheat the oven to 300°F.

2. Grind the flaxseed in an electric coffee grinder. Pour the ground seeds into a medium-size mixing bowl. Add the whole-wheat pastry flour, sugar, soy flour, cocoa powder, and baking powder. Stir with a wire whisk until thoroughly combined.

3. Pour the soy milk into a small bowl. Add the molasses and vanilla. Stir. Pour into the dry ingredients. Stir to form a batter. Continue stirring until the batter bubbles and thickens.

4. Spoon 2-tablespoon-size mounds of cookie batter onto a nonstick or oiled cookie sheet, about eight evenly spaced cookies on a sheet. Bake for 15 minutes, until the bottoms of the cookies are lightly browned and the cookies have a cakelike texture.

≋ SORBET

If you try to freeze tofu, it comes out crumbly—never creamy. How can you possibly make sorbet out of it? Just throw it into a food processor or blender with some frozen fruit. You get soft-serve sorbet!

CHOCOLATE-STRAWBERRY SORBET

≋

Work Time: *under 5 minutes*
Equipment: *electric blender or electric food processor*
Yield: *Makes 4 servings*

Chocolate and strawberry—the perfect cold combination.

16-ounce package frozen unsweetened strawberries
1 cake (19 ounces) silken tofu
¼ cup unsweetened cocoa powder

⅓ cup all-fruit strawberry jam
1 teaspoon orange extract
1 tablespoon vanilla extract

Place all of the ingredients in an electric blender or a food processor with the S blade inserted. Blend or process until thick and creamy. Taste. If needed, add more orange extract or vanilla. Serve immediately.

PLANT ESTROGEN ESTIMATE: **1** PORTION PER SERVING

BANANA SORBET

Work Time: *under 5 minutes*
Equipment: *electric blender or electric food processor*
Yield: *Makes 4 servings*

The frozen melon balls are a necessary ingredient. Without them, you get a creamy, cold pudding. With them, you get sorbet.

2 frozen bananas, sliced
1 cake (19 ounces) silken tofu
2 cups frozen melon balls
1 tablespoon lemon juice

1 teaspoon banana extract
1 tablespoon vanilla extract
2 tablespoons maple syrup

Place all of the ingredients in an electric blender or a food processor with the S blade inserted. Blend or process until thick and creamy. Taste. If needed, add more banana extract or vanilla. Serve immediately.

PLANT ESTROGEN ESTIMATE: **1** PORTION PER SERVING

ORANGE-GINGER SORBET

Work Time: *under 5 minutes*
Equipment: *electric blender or electric food processor*
Yield: *Makes 4 servings*

A high-C variation of ginger ice cream.

6 ⅛×1-inch slices fresh ginger
1 cake (19 ounces) silken tofu
2 cups frozen melon balls
⅓ cup frozen orange juice concentrate

2 tablespoons all-fruit orange marmalade
1 teaspoon orange extract
2 tablespoons maple syrup

Place all of the ingredients in an electric blender or a food processor with the S blade inserted. Blend or process until thick and creamy. Taste. If needed, add more orange extract. Serve immediately.

> **PLANT ESTROGEN ESTIMATE: 1 PORTION PER SERVING**

CHERRY-ALMOND SORBET

Work Time: *under 5 minutes*
Equipment: *electric blender or electric food processor*
Yield: *Makes 4 servings*

Cherries alone don't disguise the taste of tofu. They need help from almond extract.

16-ounce package frozen pitted cherries
1 cake (19 ounces) silken tofu
½ cup all-fruit cherry preserves

1 teaspoon lemon extract
1 teaspoon almond extract

Place all of the ingredients in an electric blender or a food processor with the S blade inserted. Blend or process until thick and creamy. Taste. If needed, add more lemon or almond extract. Serve immediately.

> **PLANT ESTROGEN ESTIMATE: 1 PORTION PER SERVING**

STRAWBERRY SORBET

Work Time: *under 5 minutes*
Equipment: *electric blender or electric food processor*
Yield: *Makes 4 servings*

Strawberries are a great source of boron—one of the best bone-protective minerals.

16-ounce package frozen unsweetened strawberries
1 cake (19 ounces) silken tofu

½ cup all-fruit strawberry jam
1 teaspoon vanilla extract
1 teaspoon lemon extract

Place all of the ingredients in an electric blender or a food processor with the S blade inserted. Blend or process until thick and creamy. Taste. If needed, add more vanilla or lemon extract. Serve immediately.

PLANT ESTROGEN ESTIMATE: **1** PORTION PER SERVING

Sources of Ingredients

Silk (soy milk)
White Wave, Inc.
Boulder, CO 80301

Soy Nuts, Soy Flour, and Flaxseed
Arrowhead Mills, Inc.
Box 2059
Hereford, TX 79045

Silken, Soft, Firm, and Extra-Firm Tofu
Nasoya Foods, Inc.
23 Jytek Drive
Leominister, MA 01453

Fat-Free Meat-Mimicking Products
Lightlife Foods, Inc.
Greenfield, MA 01302

High-Lignan Flax Oil
Barclean's Organic Oils
4936 Lake Terrel Road
Ferndale, WA 98248

Ready-Made Estrogenic Foods
The Estrogen Pantry
47 Summer St.
Amherst, MA 01002
www.estrogen-anaturalway.com
Fax: (413) 549–0020

References

≋ BOOKS

Beard, R. J., ed. *The Menopause: A Guide to Current Research and Practice.* Lancaster, England: MTD Press, 1976.

Carper, Jean. *Stop Aging Now!* New York: HarperCollins Publishers, 1995.

Lark, Susan M., M.D. *The Estrogen Decision.* Los Altos, Calif.: Westchester Publishing Company, 1994.

Love, Susan, M.D., with Karen Lindsey. *Dr. Susan Love's Breast Book.* New York: Addison-Wesley Publishing Company, 1991.

———. *Dr. Susan Love's Hormone Book: Making Informed Choices About Menopause.* New York: Random House, 1997.

Messina, Mark, Ph.D., Virginia Messina, R.D., and Ken Setchell, Ph.D. *The Simple Soybean and Your Health.* Garden City Park, N.Y.: Avery Publishing Group, 1994.

Northrup, Christiane, M.D. *Women's Bodies, Women's Wisdom.* New York: Bantam Books, 1994.

Notelovitz, Morris, M.D., and Diana Tonessen. *Menopause and Mid-life.* New York: St. Martin's Press, 1993.

Ojeda, Linda, Ph.D. *Menopause Without Medicine.* Alameda, Calif.: Hunter House, 1995.

Sears, Barry, and Bill Lawren. *The Zone.* New York: Regan Books, 1995.

Sheehy, Gail. *New Passages.* New York: Random House, 1993.

Somer, Elizabeth. *Nutrition for Women: The Complete Guide.* New York: Henry Holt, Inc., 1993.

Ulene, Art, M.D. *The NutriBase Nutrition Facts Desk Reference.* Garden City Park, N.Y.: Avery Publishing Group, 1995.

Weil, Andrew, M.D. *Spontaneous Healing.* New York: Alfred A. Knopf, 1995.

☰ ARTICLES

Adlercreutz, H. "Urinary Excretion of Lignans and Isoflavoid Phytoestrogens in Japanese Men and Women." *Journal of Clinical Nutrition* 54:6 (1991) 1093–1100.

———. "Diet and Breast Cancer." *Acta Oncologica* 31:2 (1992) 175–81.

———. "Dietary Phytoestrogens and the Menopause in Japan." *Lancet* 339 (May 16, 1992) 1233.

———. "Dietary Phytoestrogens and Cancer: Invitro and Invivo Studies." *Journal of Steroid Biochemistry and Molecular Biology* 41:3–8 (1992) 331–33.

———. "Lignans and Isoflavonoids of Dietary Origin and Hormone-Dependent Cancer." *Food and Cancer Prevention: Chemical and Biological Aspects* (Cambridge, England: Royal Society of Chemistry, 1993) 348–52.

———. "Inhibition of Aromatase by Mammalian Lignans and Isoflavonoid Phytoestrogens." *Journal of Steroid Biochemistry and Molecular Biology* 44:2 (1993) 147–53.

———. "Estrogen Metabolism and Excretion in Oriental and Caucasian Women." *Journal of the National Cancer Institute* 86:14 (1994) 1076–82.

———. "Determination of Lignans and Isoflavonoids in Plasma of Omnivorous and Vegetarian Women by Isotope Dilution Gas Chromatography-mass Spectrometry." *Cancer Detection and Prevention* 18:4 (1994) 259–71.

———. "Lignan and Isoflavonoid Conjugates in Human Urine." *Journal of Steroid Biochemistry and Molecular Biology* 52:1 (1995) 97–103.

———. "Soybean Phytoestrogen Intake and Cancer Risk." *Journal of Nutrition* 125 (1995) 757S–70S.

Ajuah, A. O. "Effect of Dietary Full-Fat Flaxseed With and Without Antioxidant on Fatty-Acid Composition of Major Lipid Classes of Chicken Meat." *Poultry Science* 72:1 (1993) 125–36.

Albertson, Ellen. "Super Soy: The Newest Miracle Food." *Self* (October 1995) 148–151.

Amarowicz, R. "Chromatographic Separation of Flaxseed Phenolics." *Nuhrung* 38:5 (1994) 520–26.

Anderson, D. L. "Concentrations and Intakes of H, B, S, K, Na, Cl, and NaCl in Foods." *Journal of Food Composition and Analysis* 7 (1994) 59–82.

Anderson, J. W. "Meta-Analysis of Effects of Soy Protein Intake on Serum Lipids." *New England Journal of Medicine* 333:5 (1995) 276–82.

Anthony, M. S. "Plant and Mammalian Estrogen Effects on Plasma Lipids of Female Monkeys." *Circulation* 90 (1994) Suppl. I-235 abstract.

———. "Effects of Soy Protein Phytoestrogens on Cardiovascular Risk Factors in Rhesus Monkeys." *Journal of Nutrition* 125 (1995) Suppl. 38:803s–4s abstract.

———. "Does Soy Supplementation Improve Coronary Heart Disease (CHD) Risk?" *Circulation* 91 (1995) 925 abstract.

Bambagiotti-Alberti, M. "Investigation of Mammalian Lignan Precursors in Flax Seed: first evidence of secoisolriciresinol diglucoside in two isomeric forms in liquid chromatograph/mass spectrometry." *Rapid Communication in Mass Spectrometry* 8:12 (1994) 929–32.

Barnes, S. "Soybeans Inhibit Mammary Tumor Growth Models of Breast Cancer." In *Mutagens and Carcinogens in the Diet,* M. W. Pariza, ed. (Wiley-Liss: New York, 1990) 239–53.

———. "Potential Role of Dietary Isoflavones in the Prevention of Cancer." *Advances in Experimental Medicine and Biology* 354 (1994) 135–47.

———. "Biochemical Targets of Isoflavone Genistein in Tumor Cell Lines." *Proceedings of the Society for Experimental Biology and Medicine* 208 (1995) 103–7.

———. "Effect of Genistein on Vitro and In Vivo Models of Cancer." *Journal of Nutrition* 125:3 (1995) Suppl. 777S–83S.

Bland, Jeffrey. *Applying the New Essentials in Nutritional Medicine* (Health Comm. International, Inc., 1995) tapes 3 and 4.

Bierenbaum, M. L. "Reducing Atherogenic Risk in Hyperlipemic Humans with Flaxseed Supplementation: A Preliminary Report." *Journal of the American College of Nutrition* 12:5 (1993) 501–4.

Brink, Susan. "A Drug for Fragile Bones." *U.S. News and World Report* (November 6, 1995) 89–90.

Brandi, M. L. "Flavoids: Biochemical Effects on Therapeutic Applications." *Bone and Mineral* 19 Suppl. (1992) S3–14.

Breslau, N. A. "Relationship of Animal Protein–Rich Diet to Kidney Stone Formation and Calcium Metabolism." *Journal of Clinical Endocrinology and Metabolism* 66 (1988) 140–46.

Cassidy, A. "Biological Effects of Plant Estrogens in Premenopausal Women." *American Society for Experimental Biology* (abs): A866, 1993.

Chan, J. K. "Effect of Dietary Alpha-linolenic Acid and Its Ratio to Linoleic Acid on Platelet and Plasma Fatty Acids and Thrombogenesis." *Lipids* 28:9 (1993) 811–17.

Cherian, G. "Omega-3 Fatty Acid and Cholesterol Content of Newly Hatched Chicks from Alpha-linolenic Acid–Enriched Eggs." *Lipids* 27:9 (1992) 706–10.

Chung, H. "How to Reduce Risk Factors of Osteoporosis in Asia." *Chinese Medical Journal* 55:3 (1995) 209–13.

Colditz, G. A. "The Uses of Estrogens and Progestins and the Risk of Breast Cancer in Postmenopausal women." *New England Journal of Medicine* 332:24 (1995) 1589–93.

Collins, S. C. "Age, Estrogens, and Psyche." *Clinical Obstetrics and Gynecology* 24:1 (1981) 219–29.

Cunnane, S. C. "High Alpha-linolenic Acid Flaxseed: Some Nutritional Properties in Humans." *British Journal of Nutrition* 69:2 (1993) 443–53.

———. "Nutritional Attributes of Traditional Flaxseed in Healthy Young Adults." *American Journal of Clinical Nutrition* 61:1 (1995) 62–68.

Dwyer, J. T. "Tofu and Soy Drinks Contain Phytoestrogens." *Journal of the American Dietetic Association* 94:7 (1994) 739–43.

Follingstad, A. H. "Estriol, the Forgotten Estrogen?" *Journal of the American Medical Association* 239 (1978) 29–30.

"Foods That May Prevent Breast Cancer: Soy Beans, Whole Wheat and Green Tea, Among Others." *Primary Care and Cancer* 4:2 (February 1994) 10–11.

Foreman, Judy. "Navigating the Maze of the Estrogen Replacement Debate." *The Boston Globe* (July 10, 1995) 25.

———. "In Estrogen Therapy, Is Less Better?" *The Boston Globe* (December 16, 1996) C1, C4.

Fotsis, T. "Genistein, a Dietary-Derived Inhibitor of Vitro Angiogenesis." *Proceedings of the National Academy of Sciences in the United States of America* 90:7 (1993) 2690–94.

Fukita, T. "Comparison of Osteoporosis and Calcium Intake Between Japan and the United States." *PSEBM* 200 (1992) 149–52.

Gaddi, A. "Dietary Treatment for Familial Hypercholesterolemia—Differential Effects of Dietary Soy Protein According to the Apoliprotein E Phenotypes." *American Journal of Nutrition* 53 (1991) 1191–96.

Garreau, B. "Phytoestrogens: New Ligands for Rats and Human Alpha-Fetoprotein." *Biochimica et Biophysica Acta* 1094 (1991) 339–45.

Harris, R. K. "Assays for Potentially Anticarcinogenic Phytoestrogens in Flaxseed." *Cereal Foods World* 38: 3 (1993) 147–51.

Hill, P. "Diet, Lifestyle and Menstrual Activity." *American Journal of Clinical Nutrition,* 33 (1980) 1192.

Hunt, C. D. "Concentrations of Boron and Other Elements in Human Foods and Personal Care Products." *Research* 91:5 (1991) 558–68.

Hutchins, Andrea. "Urinary Isoflavonoid, Phytoestrogen and Lignan Excretion After Consumption of Fermented and Unfermented Soy Products." *Journal of the American Dietetic Association* 95 (1995) 545–51.

———. "Vegetables, Fruits and Legumes: Effect on Urinary Isoflavonoid Phytoestrogen and Lignan Excretion." *Journal of the American Dietetic Association* 95 (1995) 769–74.

Ingram, A. J. "Effects of Flaxseed and Flax Oil Diets in Rat-5/5 Renal Ablation Model." *American Journal of Kidney Diseases* 25: 2 (1995) 320–29.

Jaroff, Leon. "The Man's Cancer," *Time* (April 1, 1996) 58–65.

Joannou, G. E. "A Urinary Profile Study of Dietary Phytoestrogens." *Journal of Steroid Biochemistry and Molecular Biology* 54:3–4 (1995) 167–84.

Kalu, D. N. "Modulation of Age-Related Hyperparathyroidism and Senile Bone Loss in Fischer Rats by Soy Protein and Food Restriction." *Endocrinology* 122 (1988) 1847–54.

Kanazawa, T. "Soy and Heart Disease Prevention." *Journal of Nutrition* 125 (1995) 639S–46S.

Kasper, R. "Biotransformation of Naturally Occurring Lignan—Arctigenin in Mammalian Cell Lines Genetically Engineered for Expression of Single Cytochrome P450 Isoforms." *Planta-Medica* 60:5 (1994) 441–44.

Kelley, D. S. "Dietary Alpha-linolenic Acid and Immunocompetence in Humans." *American Journal of Clinical Nutrition* 53:1(1991) 40–46.

Kelly, G. E. "The Variable Metabolic Response to Dietary Isoflavones in Humans." *Proceedings of the Society for Experimental Biology and Medicine* 208 (1995) 40–43.

Kennedy, Ann. "The Evidence for Soybean Products as Cancer Preventive Agents." *Journal of Nutrition* 125 (1995) 733S–34S.

Kritchevsky, D. "Atherogenicity of Animal and Vegetable Protein—Influence of Lysine to Arginine Ratio." *Atherosclerosis* 41 (1982) 429–31.

Kurzer, M. S. "Fecal Lignan and Isoflavonoid Excretion in Premenopausal Women Consuming Flaxseed Powder." *Cancer Epidemiology, Biomarkers and Prevention* 4:4 (1995) 353–58.

Laerin, Danielle. "Effects of Soy-Protein Beverage on Plasma Lipoproteins in Children with Familial Hypercholesterolemia." *American Journal of Clinical Nutrition* 54 (1991) 93–103.

Lamartiniere, Carol. "Neonatal Genistein Chemoprevents Mammary Cancer." *Proceedings of the Society for Experimental Biology and Medicine* 208 (1995) 120–23.

Lampe, J. W. "Urinary Lignan and Isoflavonoid Excretion in Premenopausal Women Consuming Flaxseed Powder." *American Journal of Clinical Nutrition* 60:1 (1994) 122–28.

Lemon, H. M. "Estriol Prevention of Mammary Carcinoma Induced by 7, 12-Dimenthylbenzanthracene and Procarbazine." *Cancer Research* 35 (1975) 1341–53.

———. "Pathophysiologic Considerations in the Treatment of Menopausal Patients with Estrogens; The Role of Estriol in Prevention of Mammary Carcinoma." *Acta Endocrinolgica* 233 Suppl. (1980) 17–27.

———. "Reduced Estriol Excretion on DMBA-Induced Breast Tumors." *Journal of Steroid Biochemistry* 20 (Rp. 1984) 1067–75.

Markavarich, B. M. "Effects of Coumestrol on Estrogen Receptor Function and Uterine Growth in Ovariectomized Rats." *Environmental Health Perspectives* 103 (6) 574–81.

Markiewicz, L. "In Vitro Bioassays of Non-steroidal Phytoestrogens." *Journal of Steroid Biochemistry and Molecular Biology* 45:5 (1993) 399–405.

McBean, Lois. "Osteoporosis: Visions for Care and Prevention—Conference Report." *Journal of the American Diabetic Association* 94 (1994): 668–71.

Melis, G. B. "Ipraflavone and Low Doses of Estrogens in the Prevention of Bone Mineral Loss in Climacterium." *Bone and Mineral* 19:S1 (1992) S49–56.

Messina, Mark. "The Role of Soy Products in Reducing Risk of Cancer." *Journal of the National Cancer Institute* 83:8 (1991) 541–45.

———. "Increasing Use of Soy Foods and Their Potential in Cancer Prevention." *The Journal of the American Dietetic Association* 91:7 (1991) 836–40.

Miksicek, R. J. "Commonly Occurring Plant Flavonoids Have Estrogenic Activity." *Molecular Pharmacology* 44:1 (1993) 37–43.

———. "Interaction of Naturally Occurring Nonsteroidal Estrogens with Expressed Recombinant Human Estrogen Receptor." *Journal of Steroid Biochemistry and Molecular Biology* 49:2–3 (1994) 153–60.

Morton, M. S. "Determination of Lignans and Isoflavones in Human Female Plasma Following Dietary Supplementation." *Journal of Endocrinology* 142 (1994) 251–59.

Mousavi, Y. "Genistein Is an Effective Stimulator of Sex Hormone–Binding Globulin in Hepatocarcinoma Human Liver Cells and Suppresses Proliferation of These Cells in Culture." *Steroids* 58:7 (1993) 301–4.

Murkies, A. L. "Dietary Flour Supplementation Decreases Post-menopausal Hot Flashes: Effect of Soy and Wheat." *Maturitas: Journal of Climacteric and Postmenopause* 21:3 (1995) 189–95.

Murphy, P. A. "Phytoestrogen Content of Processed Soybean Products." *Food Technology* (January 1982) 60–64.

Murray, M. "Menopause: Is Estrogen Necessary?" *American Journal of Natural Medicine* 2:9 (1995) 9–15.

Musey, P. I. "Effect of Diet on Lignans and Isoflavonoid Phytoestrogens in Chimpanzees." *Life Sciences* 57:7 (1995) 655–64.

Nielson, F. H. "The Saga of Boron in Food: From a Banished Food Preservative to a Beneficial Nutrient for Humans." *Current Topics in Plant Biochemistry and Physiology* 10 (1991) 274–86.

———. "Boron Enhances and Mimics Effects of Estrogen Therapy in Postmenopausal Women." *The Journal of Trace Elements in Experimental Medicine* 5 (1992) 237–46.

———. "Facts and Fallacies about Boron." *Nutrition Today* (May/June 1992) 6–12.

———. "Biochemical and Physiologic Consequences of Boron Deprivation in Humans." *Environmental Health Perspectives* 102 (1994) 59–64.

Obermeyer, W. R. "Chemical Studies of Phytoestrogens and Related Compounds in Dietary Supplements: Flax and Chaparral." *Proceedings of the Society for Experimental Biology and Medicine* 208 (1995) 6–12.

Phipps, W. R. "Effect of Flax Seed Ingestion on the Menstrual Cycle." *Journal of Clinical Endocrinology and Metabolism* 77:5 (1993) 1215–19.

Ralof, Janet. "Tamoxifen Quandary: Promising Cancer Drug May Hide a Troubling Dark Side." *Science News* 141 (April 25, 1992) 266–69.

Ranhotra, G. S. "Lipidemic Response in Rats Fed Flaxseed and Sunflower Diets." *Cereal-Chemistry* 69:6 (1992) 623–25.

———. "Lipidemic Response in Rats Fed Flaxseed Oil and Meal." *Cereal-Chemistry* 70:3 (1993) 364–66.

Recker, Robert. "Calcium Absorption and Achorhydria." *New England Journal of Medicine* 327 (1992) 1637–42.

Rose, David. "Diet, Hormones and Cancer." *Annual Review of Public Health* 14 (1993) 1–17.

Santiago, L. A. "Japanese Soybean Paste Miso Scavenges Free Radicals and Inhibits Lipid Peroxidation." *Journal of Nutrition and Vitaminology* 38 (1992) 297–304.

Sathyamoorthy, N. "Stimulation of pS2 Expression by Diet-derived Compounds." *Cancer Research* 54 (1994) 957–61.

Serraino, S. "The Effect of Flaxseed Supplementation on the Initiation and Promotional Stages of Mammary Tumorgenesis." *Nutrition and Cancer* 17-2 (1992) 153–59.

Setchell, K. "Naturally Occurring Nonsteroidal Estrogens in Dietary Origins." In *Estrogens in the Environment II: Influence on Development,* J. A. McLaclan, ed. (New York: Elsevier, 1985) 69–85.

Sharma, O. P. "Soy of Dietary Source Plays a Preventive Role Against the Pathogenesis of Prostatitis in Rats." *Journal of Steroid Biochemistry and Molecular Biology* 43:6 (1992) 557–64.

Sirtori, C. R. "Soybean Protein Diet and Plasma Cholesterol: From Therapy to Molecular Mechanisms." *Annals of the New York Academy of Sciences* 678 (1993) 188–201.

———. "Soybean-Protein Diet in the Treatment of Type II Hyperlipoproteinaemia." *Lancet* 5 (1997) 275–77.

Steele, V. E. "Cancer Chemoprevention Agent Development Strategies for Genistein." *Journal of Nutrition* 125: 3S (1995) 713S–16S.

Thompson, Lillian. "Mammalian Lignan Production from Various Foods." *Nutrition and Cancer* 16:1 (1991) 43–51.

———. "Potential Health Benefits and Problems Associated with Antinutrients in Foods." *Food Research International* 26: 2 (1993) 131–49.

Von Schacky, Clemon. "Prophylax of Atherosclerosis with Marine Omega-3 Fatty Acids." *Annals of Internal Medicine* 107 (1987) 890–99.

Wallis, Claudia. "The Estrogen Dilemma." *Time* (June 26, 1995) 46–53.

Wang, C. "Lignans and Flavonoids Inhibit Aromatase Enzyme in Human Preadipocytes." *Journal of Steroid Biochemistry and Molecular Biology* 50:3–4 (1994) 205–12.

Wang, H. "Isoflavone Content in Commercial Soy Foods." *Journal of Agriculture and Food Chemistry* 42 (1994) 1666–73.

Wei, Huachen. "Antioxidant and Antipromotional Effects of Soybean Isoflavone Genistein." *Proceedings of the Society for Experimental Biology and Medicine* 208 (1995) 4–7.

Whitaker, Julian. "Preventing Breast Cancer." *Health and Healing* (January 1994, supplement).

Wilcox, G. "Oestrogenic Effects of Plant Foods on Postmenopausal Women." *British Medical Journal* 301 (1991) 905–6.

Wotiz, H. H., Beebe, D. R., and Muller, E. "Effect of Estrogens on DMBA-Induced Breast Tumors." *Journal of Steroid Biochemistry* 20 (1984) 1067–75.

Ziegler, Jan. "Just the Flax, Ma'am: Researchers Testing Linseed." *Journal of the National Cancer Institute* 86:23 (1994) 1746–49.

General Index

A

Adlercreutz, Herman, xxvi
adrenal glands, xviii

B

Baird, Donna, xxxii
Barnes, Stephen, xxiii, xxiv, xxxii, 34
Bierenbaum, M. L., xxix
bladder cancer, xxiii
Bland, Jeffrey, xxiv–xxv
blood clotting, xvi
Bock, Martin, 6
bones, 42
    preservation of, xv, xxx–xxxiii, 10
    see also osteoporosis
boron, xxxi, xxxii, 36–37, 42–43, 161
breast cancer, xxviii, 3, 17–18
    fat intake and, xxv, 14
    overweight and, xix, 8
    plant estrogen dose and, 16, 22
    protection against, xvi–xix, xxii–xxvii,
        xxxii, xxxiii, 8, 10
    risk factors for, xv, xvi, xviii, xix, xx, xxx,
        8–9
Breslau, Neil, xxx

C

calcium, xxx, xxxi, 6, 28
cancers, xvi–xvii, xviii–xx
    protection against, xxii–xxiv, xxvi, xxxii,
        10, 24
    see also breast cancer
cardiovascular disease. *See* heart disease
cardiovascular health, plant estrogen dose
    and, 22
Cassidy, A., xxiv
cholesterol, xxviii–xxix, xxxii, xxxiii, 10, 14,
    24
    plant estrogen dose and, 16,
        22–23
Colditz, Graham, xx
Colgan, Michael, 24
colon cancer, xxiii, xxvi
copper, xxxii
Cunnane, S. C., xxix

D

daidzein, xxiii, xxxi
dairy products, xxx, xxxi,
    13
diabetes, xvi

E

endometriosis, xvi
esophageal cancer, xxiii
estradiol, xviii–xix, xx, xxvi, xxvii, 8, 9
estriol, xviii, xix, 8
estrogen, xv–xx
  bone preservation and, xv, xxx
  as cancer promoter vs. cancer protection,
    xviii–xx
  different forms of, xvii–xix, 8
  heart protection and, xv, xix
  need for, xv
  pharmaceutical, approximating standard
    dose of, 23
  risks associated with, xv, xvi, xviii–xx, 8–9
  see also plant estrogens
estrogen pills. See hormone replacement
    therapy
estrone, xviii–xix, xx, xxvi, xxvii, 8, 9
exercise, xxxi, xxxiii, 6

F

family food, 24
fat cells, xviii, xix, xxvi, 8
fat intake, xxix
  appropriate level of, 14–15
  breast cancer and, xxv, 14
  in estrogenic diet, 11–14
fatty acids, essential, xxv, xxix, 14, 15
flax powder, 38–39
flaxseed, xvi, xvii, xx–xxii, xxxi, xxxiv, 15,
    24, 36–38, 42–43
  author's explorations into, 7, 9–11
  baking and cooking with, 21, 37–38
  breast cancer protection and, xxiv–xxvii,
    xxxiii
  dose of, xxxii, xxxiii, 16–17
  estrogenic potency of, 37
  fat calories in, 11–14
  heart protection and, xxvii–xxviii, xxix
  nutritional content of, 36–37
  reaping potential benefits of, 19
  source for, 273
flaxseed oil, xxix, 39–40, 273
Forman, Judy, 6

G

Gaddi, A., xxviii
gallbladder disease, xvi
genistein, xxiii, xxiv

H

heart attacks, xxvii–xxviii
heart disease, xvi
  fat intake and, 14
  protection against, xv, xix, xxvii–xxix
high blood pressure, xvi
hormone replacement therapy, xix–xx, xxvii,
    xxxiii–xxxiv, 3–4, 5, 16–17, 18
  alternatives to, xvii, 6–11
  bone preservation and, xv, xvi, xix, xxx, xxxi
  heart protection and, xv, xvi, xix
  risks associated with, xv, xvi, xviii, xix, 9
  side effects of, xxxiv, 4
Hutchins, Andrea, 35

I

Ipriflavone, xxxi
isoflavones, xvi, xxxi, 37
  see also plant estrogens

J

Japanese diet, xxii, 6, 7

K

Kalu, Dike, xxxi

L

Lark, Susan, xvi, xxii
Lawren, Bill, 14
lecithin, xxiii, xxviii
Lee, H. P., xxiii
Lemon, H. P., xix
lignans, xvi, xxv–xxvi, 37, 39
  see also plant estrogens
liver, xviii–xix
liver cancer, xxiii
liver disease, xvi
Love, Susan, 17–18
lung cancer, xxiii

M

magnesium, xxxii
manganese, xxxii
meat, xxx, 13
"meats," soy, 12, 34, 273
menopausal symptoms:
  alleviated by plant estrogens, xxi, xxii,
    xxvii, xxxii, xxxiii, 10
  author's experiences of, 3–6, 24–26
  plant estrogen dose and, 16, 22

menopause, estrogen production and, xviii
menstrual cycle, length of, xxiv, xxvi
Messina, Mark, xxiii, xxxi, xxxii, 36
Messina, Virginia, xxxi
Milis, G. B., xxxii
milk, xxxi, 13
miso, 35
Morton, M. S., xxi
Murikis, A. L., xxi

N

Neilson, Forrest, 36–37, 42–43, 161
Northrup, Christiane, xx, 18

O

Obermeyer, W. R., xxxiii
Ojeda, Linda, 14–15
omega-3 essential fatty acids, xxv, xxix, 14,
    15
osteoporosis, xv, xvi, xvii, xix, xxvii,
    xxx–xxxiii
    plant estrogen dose and, 16–17
ovaries, xviii
overweight, xix, 8

P

pancreatic cancer, xxiii
pantry items, 27–40
    sources for, 273
phenolic acid, xxiii
Phipps, William, xxvi
phytate, xxiii
phytoestrogens, xvi
    see also plant estrogens
phytosterols, xxiii, xxviii–xxix
plant estrogens, xx–xxxv
    author's explorations into, 7–11
    author's menopausal symptoms and,
        24–26
    author's personal program for, 21–22
    bone preservation and, xxxi, xxxiii
    cancer protection and, xvi, xvii, xviii,
        xxii–xxvii, xxxii, 8, 10
    cooking with, 19–21, 27–40
    dose of, xxxii–xxxiii, 16–17
    fat calories in, 11–14
    heart protection and, xxvii–xxix
    pantry for, 27–40
    pluses and minuses of, 15–16
    reaping potential benefits of, 18–19

recipes with most, per serving, 23
    see also flaxseed; soy
Premarin, 9
progesterone, xvi, xix, xx, xxvi, xxx, xxxiv
prostate cancer, xxiii, xxvi, 24
protease inhibitors, xxiii
protein, xxx

S

saponins, xxviii–xix
Sass, Lorna J., 37
Sathymoorthy, Neerja, xxii
Schiff, Isaac, xvi
Sears, Barry, 14
Serraino, M., xxvi
Setchell, Ken, xxiii, xxxi
Sheehy, Gail, xxx, 6
Silk, 3, 273
skin, essential oils and, 15
skin cancer, xxiii
soy, xvi, xvii, xx–xxiv, xxxiv, 6, 7
    author's explorations into, 7, 9–11
    bone preservation and, xxx–xxxiii
    cancer protection and, xvi, xxii–xxiv,
        xxvi–xxvii, xxxii, 24
    components of, xxiii
    cooking with, 28–36
    dose of, xxxii–xxxiii, 16–17
    fat calories in, 11–14
    heart protection and, xxvii–xxix
    reaping potential benefits of, 18
soybeans, 15
    whole, 31–32
soy fiber, xxviii
soy flour, 12, 33, 273
soy "meats," 12, 34, 273
soy milk, xxii–xxiii, 12, 32–33, 36, 273
soy nuts, 12, 32, 273
soy protein powders, 35–36
soy supplements, 35–36
stomach cancer, xxiii

T

tamoxifen, xxiv
tempeh, 34–35
Thompson, Lillian, xxv, xxvi
tofu, xxii–xxiii, xxxi, 6, 7, 12, 14,
    36
    cooking with, 20–21, 28–31
    extra-firm, 30–31, 273

tofu *(cont'd)*:
  firm, 30, 273
  nutritional content of, 28
  silken, 29, 273
  soft, 29–30, 273
  source for, 273
  storing, 29
tofu products, 31
TVP (texturized vegetable protein),
  34

U

uterine cancer, xix
uterine fibroid tumors, xvi

V

vitamin K, xxxii
vitamin supplementation, xxxi–xxxii, xxxiii

W

Wallace, Claudia, xxxiv
weight:
  estrogenic diet and, 11–14
  and health risks of overweight, xix, 8
Weil, Andrew, xxvii, 37
wrinkles, 15

Z

zinc, xxxii

Recipe Index

A

Almond(s):
  apricot muffins, 120
  cherry sorbet, 270
  coffee custard, 240–41
  date-nut granola, 76
  maple creamy syrup, 89
  milk, quick, 62
  shake, 67
Almost coffee by the mug, 62–63
Angel hair pasta, smoked tomato creme
    sauce over, 193
Anise:
  -and-apple Waldorf salad, 171
  and carrot in creamy sauce, 178
Apple(s):
  -and-anise Waldorf salad, 171
  bars, 46–47
  cinnamon, and malted nuts, 55
  cinnamon sauce, 232
  crumble, quick, 245
  dried, in peanut butter–nut bars, 50–51
  -molasses-nut snack bars, 44–45
  orange blintzes, 95–96
  orange pancakes, 86–87
  -raisin-spice muffins, 121

soup, curried, 135–36
torte, 249–50
Apricot(s):
  almond muffins, 120
  dried, in peanut butter–nut bars, 50–51
  dried, in trail mix, 58
  orange bars, 47–48
Artichoke(s):
  dip, 114
  hot, in lemon sauce, 176–77
Asparagus:
  crêpes, 221–22
  with lemon-garlic sauce, 179–80
  lemon risotto, 200–201
Avocado:
  cilantro dressing, 165–66
  with greens, 170
  guacamole, 110
  soup, 135

B

Bacin (bits):
  —and—black bean soup, Mexican-style,
    144
  -and-spinach omelet, 105
  tomato dressing, 162–63

Balls:
  Swedish "meatballs," 206–7
  sweet-and-sour, 211
Banana:
  frosty shake, 71–72
  nut mini-muffins, 122
  sorbet, 269
  strawberry sauce, 234–35
Bars. *See* Snack bars
Basil:
  cucumber salad, 175
  fresh, dressing, 165
  fresh, marinade, tomatoes with, 172
  pesto spread, 108–9
  –and–roasted red pepper sauce, broiled
    bluefish with, 223–24
  sauce, poached cod in, 225–26
Bean(s):
  black, –and–bacin soup, Mexican-style, 144
  chili with, 207
  green, sun-dried tomatoes, and walnuts,
    179
  soup, Tuscan, 149
  white, roasted garlic, and sausage soup,
    142
Beets, in borscht, 141
Beverages, cold. *See* Shakes
Beverages, hot, 60–64
  almost coffee by the mug, 62–63
  East Indian–style spiced milk or tea, 64
  quick almond milk, 62
  simply spiced mugfuls, 61
  spiced hot milk by the quart, 63
Bisques:
  basic, 143
  chilled tomato, 133
  curried pumpkin, 138
Black bean–and–bacin soup, Mexican-style,
  144
Blintzes:
  apple-orange, 95–96
  peach-pecan, 96–97
Blueberry:
  lemon pancakes, 83–84
  soup with strawberries, 137
Bluefish:
  broiled, with roasted red pepper–and–
    basil sauce, 223–24
  pâté, 112
Borscht, 141
Bow ties, baby peas, and salmon, 192

Breads, quick, 123–25
  brown, 125
  corn, 124
  date-nut, 123
  see also Crackers; Muffins
Breads, yeast, 125–31
  caraway-rye, 126–27
  cardamom rolls, 128–29
  cinnamon-raisin, 129–30
  pecan sticky buns, 130–31
  whole-wheat, 127–28
Breakfast fare, 73–105
  apple-orange blintzes, 95–96
  basic crêpes, 91
  cherry-filled crêpes with creamy cherry
    sauce, 92–93
  peach-pecan blintzes, 96–97
  strawberry crêpes, 93–94
  see also Breads, quick; Breads, yeast;
    Cereals, cold; Cereals, hot; Muffins;
    Pancakes; Scrambles; Snack bars
Brittles:
  cinnamon-molasses-nut bars, 53
  peanut crisps, 52
Brown bread, 125
Brownies, 262–63
Brown-rice cereal, 82
Buckwheat pancakes, 85

C

Cajun dishes and flavors:
  gumbo, 140–41
  pepper, 154–55
Cakes. *See* Cheesecakes; Mousse cakes
Caraway:
  rye bread, 126–27
  rye crackers, 116–17
Cardamom:
  custard with maple-nut sauce, 239–40
  oatmeal, creamy, 82
  rolls, 128–29
Carrot(s):
  and anise in creamy sauce, 178
  ginger soup, 146–47
  loaves, mini, 180
  orange and green pâté, 182
  orange salad, nutty, 173
  pea pods, and nuts in sweet ginger glaze,
    177
Cauliflower curry, yellow, 203–4

Cereals, cold, 74–78
    cinnamon-malt granola, 77
    date-nut granola, 76
    malted cinnamon crunch, 75–76
    maple-nut crunch, 74–75
    New England maple-cranberry granola,
        78
Cereals, hot, 78–82
    brown-rice, 82
    cracked-wheat, 81
    creamed rice, 80
    creamed wheat, 80–81
    creamy cardamom oatmeal, 82
    simple sprinkle for, 79
    transforming into estrogenic meal,
        78–79
Cheesecakes, 251–53
    lemon–poppy seed, 252–53
    orange, 251–52
Cherry:
    almond sorbet, 270
    crumble, quick, 243
    -filled crêpes with creamy cherry sauce,
        92–93
    frosty shake, 69–70
    mousse cake, 256–57
Chili:
    with beans, 207
    nouveau, 208
    nutty, 209
Chinese dishes and flavors:
    family-style tofu, 212–13
    foo yong, 217
    ginger soy sauce, 157
    tofu with shiitake mushrooms and greens,
        213
Chocolate:
    bars, crispy, 54
    brownies, 262–63
    chip–peppermint pudding, 236
    cookies, soft, 267
    frosty frappe, 71
    mousse cake with raspberry sauce, 255–56
    orange mousse cake, 258–59
    shake, 68
    snack bars, 49–50
    strawberry sorbet, 268
    velvet pudding, 235
Chowders:
    corn, 148
    New England fish, 138–39

Cilantro:
    avocado dressing, 165–66
    linguine tossed with roasted garlic and,
        191
Cinnamon:
    apples and malted nuts, 55
    apple sauce, 232
    basic bisque, 143
    coffee shake, 66–67
    crunch, malted, 75–76
    malt granola, 77
    -molasses-nut bars, 53
    raisin bread, 129–30
    sesame sauce, 231
Cod:
    New England fish chowder, 138–39
    in orange-ginger sauce, 228
    poached, in basil sauce, 225–26
Coffee:
    almond custard, 240–41
    almost, by the mug, 62–63
    cinnamon shake, 66–67
Condiments, 150–60
    nut butter, 222–23
    see also Peppers; Salts; Sauces, seasoning
Cookies, 264–67
    ginger snaps, 264–65
    lemon lace, 265–66
    oatmeal-raisin, 266–67
    soft chocolate, 267
Corn:
    bread, 124
    chowder, 148
    crackers, 117
    creamed, 185
    puffed, ball trail mix, 59
Cracked-wheat cereal, 81
Crackers, 115–18
    corn, 117
    flax, 115–16
    rye-caraway, 116–17
    tortilla bowl, 118
Cranberry(ies):
    dried, in trail mix, 58
    maple granola, New England, 78
    salad, creamy, 173–74
    snack bars, 45–46
Creamed:
    corn, 185
    potatoes, 183
Cream of rice, 80

Cream of wheat, 80–81
Crêpes, 90–94, 219–21
asparagus, 221–22
basic, 91
basic dinner, 219
cherry-filled, with creamy cherry sauce,
92–93
mushroom, 220
strawberry, 93–94
Crumbles, 242–47
apple, quick, 245
cherry, quick, 243
rhubarb, quick, 244
rhubarb custard, 247
strawberry-rhubarb, 246
Crunchy paprika, 155–56
Crustless mushroom quiche, 214–15
Cucumber:
basil salad, 175
soup, cold creamy, 134
Curry(ied)(ies), 202–5
apple soup, 135–36
mayonnaise, 108
mushroom custard, 218
nuts, sweet, 57
pumpkin bisque, 138
rice with peas, 201
salt, 153
sauce, 156
spinach, 203
Thai-style yellow, 204–5
watercress, creamy, flounder on bed of, 227
yellow cauliflower, 203–4
Custard (savory), curried mushroom, 218
Custards (sweet), 239–42
almond-coffee, 240–41
cardamom, with maple-nut sauce,
239–40
lemon, 241
pumpkin, 237
rhubarb, crumble, 247

D
Date(s):
nut bread, 123
nut breakfast bars, 43–44
nut granola, 76
nut squares, chewy, 261–62
trail mix, 58
Desserts, 230–71
brownies, 262–63

chewy date-nut squares, 261–62
gingerbread, 263–64
lemon–poppy seed cheesecake, 252–53
orange cheesecake, 251–52
pear mousse pie, 259–60
raspberry mousse, 260–61
see also Cookies; Crumbles; Custards
(sweet); Mousse cakes; Puddings; Sorbets; Tortes
Dessert sauces, 231–34
apple-cinnamon, 232
banana-strawberry, 234–35
cinnamon-sesame, 231
creamy orange, 233
creamy vanilla, 232–33
maple-nut, 239–40
peach, 234
raspberry, 255–56
Dijon (mustard):
sauce, broiled salmon with, 225
smoked mackerel sauce with fettucine,
190
vinaigrette, 167
vinaigrette, lightly creamy, 164
Dill:
garlic sauce, flounder with, 224
salt, 152
sweet potato soup, 147
vinaigrette, creamy, 162
Dips, 109–11
artichoke, 114
guacamole, 110
hummus, 110–11
Dressings. See Salad dressings

E
East Indian–style spiced milk or tea, 64
Eggplant and penne in red pepper sauce, 187

F
Family-style tofu, 212–13
Fennel. See Anise
Festive nog, 65
Fettuccine, smoked mackerel–Dijon sauce
with, 190
Fish, 222–29
bluefish pâté, 112
breaded sole with nut butter, 222–23
broiled bluefish with roasted red
pepper–and–basil sauce, 223–24
broiled salmon with Dijon sauce, 225

chowder, New England, 138–39
cod in orange-ginger sauce, 228
flounder on bed of creamy curried water-
    cress, 227
flounder with garlic-dill sauce, 224
mackerel-and-onion quiche, 215
mackerel scramble, 100
poached cod in basil sauce, 225–26
salmon, bow ties, and baby peas, 192
salmon loaf with white sauce, 228–29
smoked mackerel–Dijon sauce with fet-
    tuccine, 190
smoked mackerel pâté, 114–15
Flax(seed):
    bars, 42–54; see also Snack bars
    cold cereals, 74–78; see also Cereals, cold
    cookies and squares, 261–67; see also
        Cookies; Squares
    crackers, 115–18; see also Crackers
    lemon dressing, 166–67
    muffins and quick breads, 118–25; see also
        Breads, quick; Muffins
    nutty snacks, 54–60; see also Nutty snacks
    rice dishes with, 197–201; see also Risotto
    salts and peppers, 150–56; see also Pep-
        pers; Salts
    simple cereal sprinkle, 79
    tortes and crumbles, 242–51; see also
        Crumbles; Tortes
    yeast breads, 125–31; see also Breads, yeast
Flounder:
    on bed of creamy curried watercress, 227
    with garlic-dill sauce, 224
Foo yong, 217
Frappes:
    chocolate frosty, 71
    orange, 72
    strawberry frosty, 70
French dishes and flavors:
    spinach potage, 145–46
    vichyssoise, 133–34
Fruity syrup, creamy, 88

G
Garlic:
    dill sauce, flounder with, 224
    lemon sauce, asparagus with, 179–80
    -and-onion scramble, 98
    roasted, linguine tossed with cilantro and,
        191
    roasted, spread, 109

roasted, white bean, and sausage soup, 142
and roasted red pepper pâté, 111
sour creme, 160
Gavin's tapioca pudding, 238
Ginger:
    carrot soup, 146–47
    glaze, sweet, pea pods, carrots, and nuts
        in, 177
    orange sauce, cod in, 228
    orange sorbet, 269–70
    sauce, lightly creamy, 157
    shake, 68
    snaps, 264–65
    soy sauce, 157
Gingerbread, 263–64
Granolas:
    cinnamon-malt, 77
    date-nut, 76
    New England maple-cranberry, 78
Gravy, guilt-free, 159
Greek-style lemon soup, 139–40
Green beans, sun-dried tomatoes, and
    walnuts, 179
Greens:
    avocado with, 170
    tofu with shiitake mushrooms and, 213
Guacamole, 110
Gumbo, Cajun-style, 140–41

H
Herb:
    salt, 152–53
    vinaigrette, 168
Hummus, 110–11

I
Indian flavors:
    basic bisque, 143
    spinach potage, 145–46
    yellow cauliflower curry, 203–4
Indian pudding, 239
Israeli salad, 174–75

K
Kiwi-strawberry torte, 248–49
Kugel, noodle, 242

L
Latkes, potato, 184
Lemon:
    asparagus risotto, 200–201

Lemon *(con't)*:
　blueberry pancakes, 83–84
　custard, 241
　flaxseed dressing, 166–67
　garlic sauce, asparagus with, 179–80
　lace cookies, 265–66
　poppy seed cheesecake, 252–53
　sauce, hot artichokes in, 176–77
　soup, Greek-style, 139–40
Linguine tossed with cilantro and
　roasted garlic, 191

M

Mackerel:
　-and-onion quiche, 215
　scramble, 100
　smoked, Dijon sauce with fettuccine, 190
　smoked, pâté, 114–15
Main dishes, 202–29
　asparagus crêpes, 221–22
　basic dinner crêpes, 219
　bow ties, baby peas, and salmon, 192
　breaded sole with nut butter, 222–23
　broiled bluefish with roasted red
　　pepper–and–basil sauce, 223–24
　broiled salmon with Dijon sauce, 225
　chili with beans, 207
　cod in orange-ginger sauce, 228
　crustless mushroom quiche, 214–15
　curried mushroom custard, 218
　eggplant and penne in red pepper sauce,
　　187
　family-style tofu, 212–13
　flounder on bed of creamy curried water-
　　cress, 227
　flounder with garlic-dill sauce, 224
　foo yong, 217
　mackerel-and-onion quiche, 215
　mushroom crêpes, 220
　mushroom stroganoff, 196
　nouveau chili, 208
　nutty chili, 209
　penne and sausage in creamy tomato
　　sauce, 194
　poached cod in basil sauce, 225–26
　potato-and-pepper stew, 208–9
　salmon loaf with white sauce, 228–29
　shiitake mushroom ring with gravy, 210
　smoked mackerel–Dijon sauce with
　　fettuccine, 190

spinach curry, 203
spinach quiche, 216
Swedish "meatballs," 206–7
sweet-and-sour balls, 211
Thai-style noodles, 197
Thai-style yellow curry, 204–5
tofu with shiitake mushrooms and greens,
　213
yellow cauliflower curry, 203–4
Malt(ed):
　cinnamon crunch, 75–76
　cinnamon granola, 77
　nuts, cinnamon apples and, 55
　popcorn and nuts, 56
Maple:
　almond creamy syrup, 89
　cranberry granola, New England, 78
　nut crunch, 74–75
　nuts, 60
　nut sauce, cardamom custard with,
　　239–40
　nut syrup, 90
　walnut pudding, 236–37
Mayonnaise:
　all-purpose, 107
　curried, 108
"Meatballs," Swedish, 206–7
"Meaty" main dishes:
　chili with beans, 207
　nouveau chili, 208
　nutty chili, 209
　potato-and-pepper stew, 208–9
　shiitake mushroom ring with gravy, 210
　Swedish "meatballs," 206–7
　sweet-and-sour balls, 211
Mexican dishes and flavors:
　black bean–and–bacin soup, 144
　guacamole, 110
　omelet, 104
Middle Eastern dishes and flavors:
　hummus, 110–11
　tahini sauce, 158
Molasses:
　-apple-nut snack bars, 44–45
　brown bread, 125
　-cinnamon-nut bars, 53
　cream syrup, 89–90
　Indian pudding, 239
Mousse(s), 253–61
　pear, pie, 259–60

raspberry, 260–61
Mousse cakes, 253–59
  cherry, 256–57
  chocolate, with raspberry sauce, 255–56
  chocolate-orange, 258–59
  orange, 254–55
Muffins, 118–22
  almond-apricot, 120
  apple-raisin-spice, 121
  banana-nut mini-, 122
  orange–poppy seed, 119–20
Munchables, 41–72
  see also Beverages, hot; Nutty snacks;
    Shakes; Snack bars
Mung bean sprouts:
  foo yong, 217
  Thai-style noodles, 197
Mushroom(s):
  crêpes, 220
  custard, curried, 218
  portobello, soup, 145
  quiche, crustless, 214–15
  risotto, 199–200
  shiitake, pâté, 113
  shiitake, ring with gravy, 210
  shiitake, tofu with greens and, 213
  stroganoff, 196
  wild-, omelet, 102–3
Mustard. *See* Dijon

N

New England dishes and flavors:
  fish chowder, 138–39
  maple-cranberry granola, 78
Nog, festive, 65
Noodle(s):
  with creamy sesame sauce, 195
  kugel, 242
  mushroom stroganoff over, 196
  Thai-style, 197
Nouveau chili, 208
Nut:
  butter, 222–23
  date bread, 123
  date breakfast bars, 43–44
  date granola, 76
  date squares, chewy, 261–62
  maple crunch, 74–75
  maple sauce, cardamom custard with,
    239–40

maple syrup, 90
peachy pecan bars, 48–49
pecan-peach blintzes, 96–97
see also Soy nut(s)
Nutty chili, 209
Nutty snacks, 54–60
  cinnamon apples and malted nuts, 55
  malted popcorn and nuts, 56
  maple nuts, 60
  puffed corn ball trail mix, 59
  sweet curried nuts, 57
  trail mix, 58

O

Oat(meal)(s):
  cinnamon-malt granola, 77
  creamy cardamom, 82
  date-nut granola, 76
  New England maple-cranberry granola, 78
  pancakes, Swedish, 84
  raisin cookies, 266–67
Okra, in Cajun-style gumbo, 140–41
Olive–and–roasted red pepper dressing, 163
Omelets, 101–5
  basic, 102
  Mexican, 104
  spinach-and-bacin, 105
  tips for, 101
  wild-mushroom, 102–3
Onion:
  -and-garlic scramble, 98
  -and-mackerel quiche, 215
  vichyssoise, 133–34
Orange:
  apple blintzes, 95–96
  apple pancakes, 86–87
  apricot bars, 47–48
  carrot salad, nutty, 173
  cheesecake, 251–52
  chocolate mousse cake, 258–59
  dressing, sweet, 166
  frappe, 72
  ginger sauce, cod in, 228
  ginger sorbet, 269–70
  mousse cake, 254–55
  poppy seed muffins, 119–20
  sauce, creamy, 233
  shake, 66
  syrup, creamy, 88–89
Orange and green pâté, 182

Orzo with roasted red pepper–and–watercress sauce, 189

P

Pancakes, 83–87
  apple-orange, 86–87
  buckwheat, 85
  lemon-blueberry, 83–84
  oatmeal, Swedish, 84
  potato latkes, 184
  rice-wheat, 86
Pancake syrups. *See* Syrups
Paprika, crunchy, 155–56
Pasta, 186–97
  angel hair, smoked tomato creme sauce over, 193
  bow ties, baby peas, and salmon, 192
  eggplant and penne in red pepper sauce, 187
  linguine tossed with cilantro and roasted garlic, 191
  orzo with roasted red pepper–and–watercress sauce, 189
  penne and sausage in creamy tomato sauce, 194
  smoked mackerel–Dijon sauce with fettuccine, 190
  sun-dried tomato and walnut toss with penne, 188
  see also Noodles
Pâtés, 109, 111–15
  bluefish, 112
  orange and green, 182
  roasted red pepper–and–garlic, 111
  shiitake mushroom, 113
  smoked mackerel, 114–15
Peach(es):
  peachy pecan bars, 48–49
  pecan blintzes, 96–97
  sauce, 234
Peanut butter–nut bars, 50–51
Peanut crisps, 52
Pear mousse pie, 259–60
Pea(s):
  baby, bow ties, and salmon, 192
  curried rice with, 201
  pods, carrots, and nuts in sweet ginger glaze, 177
Pecan:
  bar, peachy, 48–49

peach blintzes, 96–97
sticky buns, 130–31
torte, 250–51
Penne:
  and eggplant in red pepper sauce, 187
  and sausage in creamy tomato sauce, 194
  sun-dried tomato and walnut toss with, 188
Pepper (green), -and-potato stew, 208–9
Pepper, red:
  roasted, –and–basil sauce, broiled bluefish with, 223–24
  roasted, and garlic pâté, 111
  roasted, –and–olive dressing, 163
  roasted, –and–watercress sauce, orzo with, 189
  sauce, eggplant and penne in, 187
Peppers (condiments), 154–55
  Cajun, 154–55
  seedy, 155
Peppermint:
  chocolate chip pudding, 236
  shake, 69
Pesto spread, 108–9
Pie, pear mousse, 259–60
Pineapple, in Thai-style yellow curry, 204–5
Popcorn and nuts, malted, 56
Poppy seed:
  lemon cheesecake, 252–53
  orange muffins, 119–20
Portobello mushroom soup, 145
Potage, spinach, 145–46
Potato(es):
  borscht, 141
  creamed, 183
  latkes, 184
  -and-pepper stew, 208–9
  salad, 168–69
  vichyssoise, 133–34
Puddings, 235–39
  chocolate velvet, 235
  Indian, 239
  maple-walnut, 236–37
  noodle kugel, 242
  peppermint–chocolate chip, 236
  tapioca, Gavin's, 238
Puffed corn ball trail mix, 59
Pumpkin:
  bisque, curried, 138
  custard, 237

Q

Quiches, 214–16
  crustless mushroom, 214–15
  mackerel-and-onion, 215
  spinach, 216

R

Raisin(s):
  -apple-spice muffins, 121
  brown bread, 125
  cinnamon bread, 129–30
  cinnamon-malt granola, 77
  oatmeal cookies, 266–67
  sweet curried nuts, 57
  trail mix, 58
Raspberry:
  mousse, 260–61
  sauce, chocolate mousse cake with,
    255–56
Rhubarb:
  crumble, quick, 244
  custard crumble, 247
  strawberry crumble, 246
Rice, 197–201
  bars, crispy, 51
  brown-, cereal, 82
  creamed, cereal, 80
  curried, with peas, 201
  wheat pancakes, 86
Risotto, 197–201
  lemon-asparagus, 200–201
  mushroom, 199–200
  sesame, 199
  spinach–and–sun-dried tomato,
    198
Rolls, cardamom, 128–29
Romaine, watercress, and walnut salad,
    169–70
Rye:
  bread, caraway, 126–27
  crackers, caraway, 116–17

S

Salad dressings, 162–68
  avocado-cilantro, 165–66
  creamy sesame, 164
  fresh basil, 165
  lemon-flaxseed, 166–67
  roasted red pepper–and–olive, 163
  sweet orange, 166

  tomato-bacin, 162–63
  see also Vinaigrettes
Salads, 168–75
  apple-and-anise Waldorf, 171
  avocado with greens, 170
  creamy cranberry, 173–74
  cucumber-basil, 175
  Israeli, 174–75
  nutty orange-carrot, 173
  potato, 168–69
  spinach-sesame, 171–72
  tomatoes with fresh basil marinade, 172
  watercress, romaine, and walnut,
    169–70
Salmon:
  bow ties, and baby peas, 192
  broiled, with Dijon sauce, 225
  loaf with white sauce, 228–29
Salsa-and-sausage scramble, 99
Salts, 150–54
  curry, 153
  dill, 152
  flax, 151
  herb, 152–53
  sesame, 150–51
  Thai, 154
Sandwich spreads. *See* Spreads
Satay sauce, creamy, 158
Sauces:
  basil, 226
  creamy cherry, 92–93
  roasted red pepper–and–basil, 223–24
  sweet-and-sour, 211
  white, 229
  see also Dessert sauces
Sauces, seasoning, 156–60
  creamy satay, 158
  curry, 156
  garlic sour creme, 160
  ginger soy, 157
  guilt-free gravy, 159
  lightly creamy ginger, 157
  tahini, 158
Sausage, soy:
  Cajun-style gumbo, 140–41
  and penne in creamy tomato sauce, 194
  roasted garlic, and white bean soup, 142
  -and-salsa scramble, 99
Scrambles, 97–101
  garlic-and-onion, 98

Scrambles *(con't)*:
  mackerel, 100
  salsa-and-sausage, 99
  veggie, 100–101
Seedy pepper, 155
Sesame:
  cinnamon sauce, 231
  dressing, creamy, 164
  risotto, 199
  salt, 150–51
  sauce, creamy, noodles with, 195
  spinach salad, 171–72
Shakes, 64–72
  almond, 67
  banana frosty, 71–72
  cherry frosty, 69–70
  chocolate, 68
  chocolate frosty frappe, 71
  cinnamon-coffee, 66–67
  festive nog, 65
  ginger, 68
  orange, 66
  orange frappe, 72
  peppermint, 69
  strawberry frosty frappe, 70
Shiitake mushroom(s):
  pâté, 113
  ring with gravy, 210
  tofu with greens and, 213
Side dishes:
  curried rice with peas, 201
  lemon-asparagus risotto, 200–201
  linguine tossed with cilantro and roasted
    garlic, 191
  mushroom risotto, 199–200
  noodles with creamy sesame sauce, 195
  orzo with roasted red pepper–and–water-
    cress sauce, 189
  sesame risotto, 199
  smoked tomato creme sauce over angel
    hair pasta, 193
  spinach–and–sun-dried tomato risotto,
    198
  sun-dried tomato and walnut toss with
    penne, 188
  see also Vegetable side dishes
Simply spiced mugfuls, 61
Snack bars, 42–54
  apple, 46–47
  chocolate, 49–50
  cinnamon-molasses-nut, 53

  cranberry, 45–46
  crispy chocolate, 54
  crispy rice, 51
  date-nut breakfast, 43–44
  molasses-apple-nut, 44–45
  orange-apricot, 47–48
  peachy pecan, 48–49
  peanut butter–nut, 50–51
  peanut crisps, 52
Snacks, 41–72
  see also Beverages, hot; Nutty snacks;
    Shakes; Snack bars
Sole, breaded, with nut butter, 222–23
Sorbets, 268–71
  banana, 269
  cherry-almond, 270
  chocolate-strawberry, 268
  orange-ginger, 269–70
  strawberry, 271
Soups, chilled, 132–37
  avocado, 135
  blueberry, with strawberries, 137
  creamy cucumber, 134
  creamy strawberry, 136
  curried apple, 135–36
  tomato bisque, 133
  vichyssoise, 133–34
Soups, hot, 137–49
  basic bisque, 143
  borscht, 141
  Cajun-style gumbo, 140–41
  corn chowder, 148
  curried pumpkin bisque, 138
  ginger-carrot, 146–47
  Greek-style lemon, 139–40
  Mexican-style black bean–and–bacin, 144
  New England fish chowder, 138–39
  portobello mushroom, 145
  roasted garlic, white bean, and sausage, 142
  spinach potage, 145–46
  sweet potato–dill, 147
  Tuscan bean, 149
Sour creme, garlic, 160
Soy "meats":
  Swedish "meatballs," 206–7
  see also Sausage, soy
Soy milk:
  hot mugs, 60–64; *see also* Beverages, hot
  shakes, 64–72; *see also* Shakes
Soy nut(s):
  cinnamon-malt granola, 77

cinnamon-molasses-nut bars, 53
malted, cinnamon apples and, 55
malted popcorn and, 56
maple, 60
molasses-apple-nut snack bars, 44–45
nutty orange-carrot salad, 173
peanut butter–nut bars, 50–51
peanut crisps, 52
pea pods, and carrots in sweet ginger
glaze, 177
puffed corn ball trail mix, 59
sweet curried, 57
Thai salt, 154
trail mix, 58
Soy sauce, ginger, 157
Spice(d):
-apple-raisin muffins, 121
hot milk by the quart, 63
milk or tea, East Indian–style, 64
simply, mugfuls, 61
Spinach:
-and-bacin omelet, 105
curry, 203
loaves, mini, 181
orange and green pâté, 182
potage, 145–46
quiche, 216
sesame salad, 171–72
and sun-dried tomato risotto, 198
tofu with shiitake mushrooms and greens,
213
Spreads, 106–9
all-purpose mayonnaise, 107
curried mayonnaise, 108
pesto, 108–9
roasted garlic, 109
see also Dips; Pâtés
Squares, 261–64
brownies, 262–63
chewy date-nut, 261–62
gingerbread, 263–64
Stews:
chili with beans, 207
nouveau chili, 208
nutty chili, 209
potato-and-pepper, 208–9
Sticky buns, pecan, 130–31
Strawberry(ies):
banana sauce, 234–35
blueberry soup with, 137
chocolate sorbet, 268

crêpes, 93–94
frosty frappe, 70
kiwi torte, 248–49
rhubarb crumble, 246
sorbet, 271
soup, creamy cold, 136
Stroganoff, mushroom, 196
Swedish dishes and flavors:
"meatballs," 206–7
oatmeal pancakes, 84
Sweet-and-sour balls, 211
Sweet curried nuts, 57
Sweet potato–dill soup, 147
Syrups, 87–90
creamy fruity, 88
creamy orange, 88–89
maple-almond creamy, 89
maple-nut, 90
molasses cream, 89–90

T

Tahini sauce, 158
Tapioca pudding, Gavin's, 238
Tea, East Indian–style spiced, 64
Thai dishes and flavors:
creamy satay sauce, 158
noodles, 197
salt, 154
yellow curry, 204–5
Tofu:
cheesecakes, 251–53; see also Cheesecakes
crêpes or blintzes, 90–97, 219–21; see also
Blintzes; Crêpes
curried mushroom custard,
218
curries, 202–5; see also Curry(ied)(ies)
dessert sauces, 231–34; see also Dessert
sauces
family-style, 212–13
foo yong, 217
mousses and mousse cakes, 253–61; see
also Mousse cakes; Mousses
omelets, 101–5; see also Omelets
pâtés and dips, 109–15; see also Dips;
Pâtés
puddings and custards, 235–42; see also
Custards (sweet); Puddings
quiches, 214–16; see also Quiches
salad dressings, 162–66; see also Salad
dressings
sauces, pasta with, 186–97; see also Pasta

Tofu (cont'd):
    scrambles, 97–101; see also Scrambles
    seasoning sauces, 156–60; see also Sauces,
      seasoning
    with shiitake mushrooms and greens, 213
    sorbets, 268–71; see also Sorbets
    soups, 132–49; see also Soups, chilled;
      Soups, hot
    spreads, 106–9; see also Spreads
    sweet-and-sour balls, 211
    vegetable side dishes with, 176–85; see
      also Vegetable side dishes
Tomato(es):
    bacin dressing, 162–63
    bisque, basic, 143
    bisque, chilled, 133
    creme sauce, smoked, over angel hair
      pasta, 193
    with fresh basil marinade, 172
    sauce, creamy, penne and sausage in, 194
Tomato(es), sun-dried:
    green beans, and walnuts, 179
    and spinach risotto, 198
    and walnut toss with penne, 188
Tortes, 248–51
    apple, 249–50
    pecan, 250–51
    strawberry-kiwi, 248–49
Tortilla bowl, 118
Trail mix, 58
    puffed corn ball, 59
Tuscan bean soup, 149
TVP (texturized vegetable protein):
    chili with beans, 207
    nouveau chili, 208
    nutty chili, 209
    potato-and-pepper stew, 208–9

V

Vanilla sauce, creamy, 232–33
Vegetable side dishes, 176–85
    asparagus with lemon-garlic sauce,
      179–80
    carrot and anise in creamy sauce, 178
    creamed corn, 185
    creamed potatoes, 183
    green beans, sun-dried tomatoes, and
      walnuts, 179
    hot artichokes in lemon sauce, 176–77

mini carrot loaves, 180
mini spinach loaves, 181
orange and green pâté, 182
pea pods, carrots, and nuts in sweet ginger
    glaze, 177
potato latkes, 184
Veggie scramble, 100–101
Vichyssoise, 133–34
Vinaigrettes:
    creamy dill, 162
    herb, 168
    lightly creamy Dijon, 164
    mustard, 167

W

Waldorf salad, apple-and-anise, 171
Walnut(s):
    chewy date-nut squares, 261–62
    chocolate snack bars, 49–50
    date-nut bread, 123
    date-nut breakfast bars, 43–44
    green beans, sun-dried tomatoes and, 179
    maple-nut crunch, 74–75
    maple-nut syrup, 90
    maple pudding, 236–37
    New England maple-cranberry granola, 78
    and sun-dried tomato toss with penne,
      188
    watercress, and romaine salad, 169–70
Watercress:
    creamy curried, flounder on bed of, 227
    –and–roasted red pepper sauce, orzo with,
      189
    romaine, and walnut salad, 169–70
    tofu with shiitake mushrooms and greens,
      213
Wheat:
    cracked-, cereal, 81
    creamed, cereal, 80–81
    rice pancakes, 86
White bean, roasted garlic, and sausage
    soup, 142
White sauce, 229
Whole-wheat bread, 127–28

Y

Yellow curries:
    cauliflower, 203–4
    Thai-style, 204–5

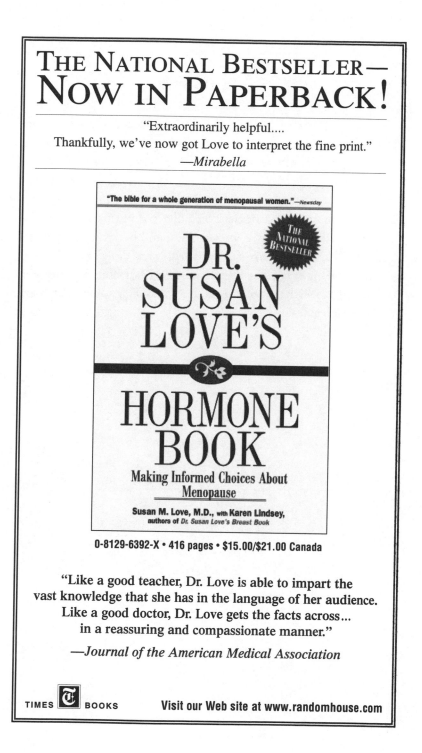

About the Author

NINA SHANDLER began writing about diet and health more than twenty years ago. Her previously published books include *The Complete Guide and Cookbook for Raising Your Child As a Vegetarian, Holiday Sweets Without Sugar, Homemade Mixes for Instant Meals the Natural Way,* and *Yoga for Pregnancy and Birth.*

For more than a decade, Shandler has been a psychologist specializing in children and families, and her articles have appeared in *The Family Therapy Networker, Teaching Tolerance,* and *Communiqué.* She lives in western Massachusetts with her husband, Michael, and daughter Sara. Her older daughter, Manju, resides in New York City.